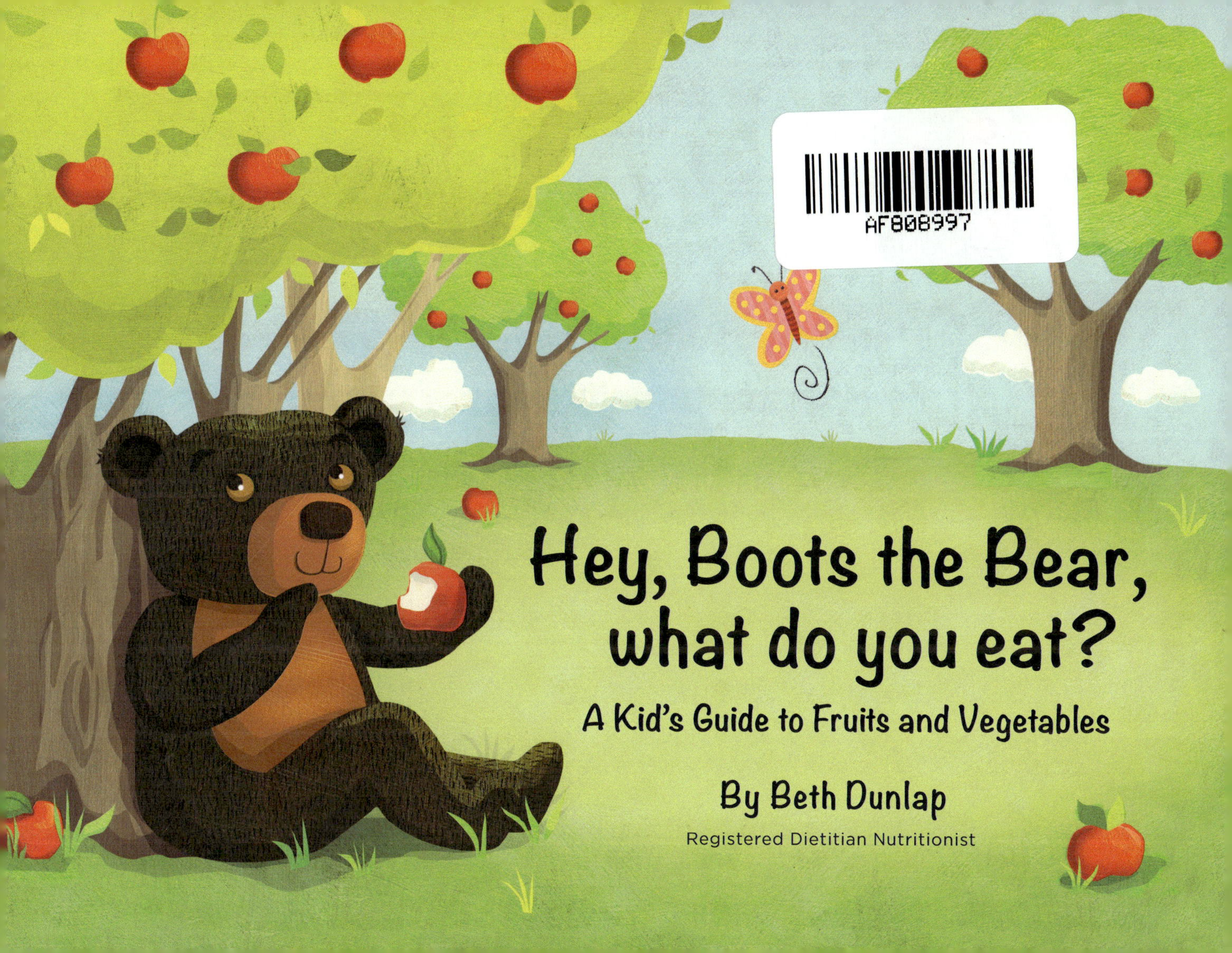

Hey, Boots the Bear, what do you eat?

A Kid's Guide to Fruits and Vegetables

By Beth Dunlap

Registered Dietitian Nutritionist

To my husband Travis
and my children Will & Andrew
whom continually support, love,
help, and encourage me!

Illustrations of Boots the Bear and Friends by Laura Watson. Book design/layout by Cheryl Casey.
Photos contributed by Beth Dunlap and Laurie Carpenter unless noted below.
Page 37 - Sontaya Chaisamutr, Shutterstock; Page 37 - Monkey Business Images, Shutterstock; Page 46 - Gan Chaonan, Shutterstock;
Page 49 - Kenishirotie, Shutterstock; Page 54 - LightField Studios, Shutterstock; Page 69 - Samuel Borges Photography, Shutterstock

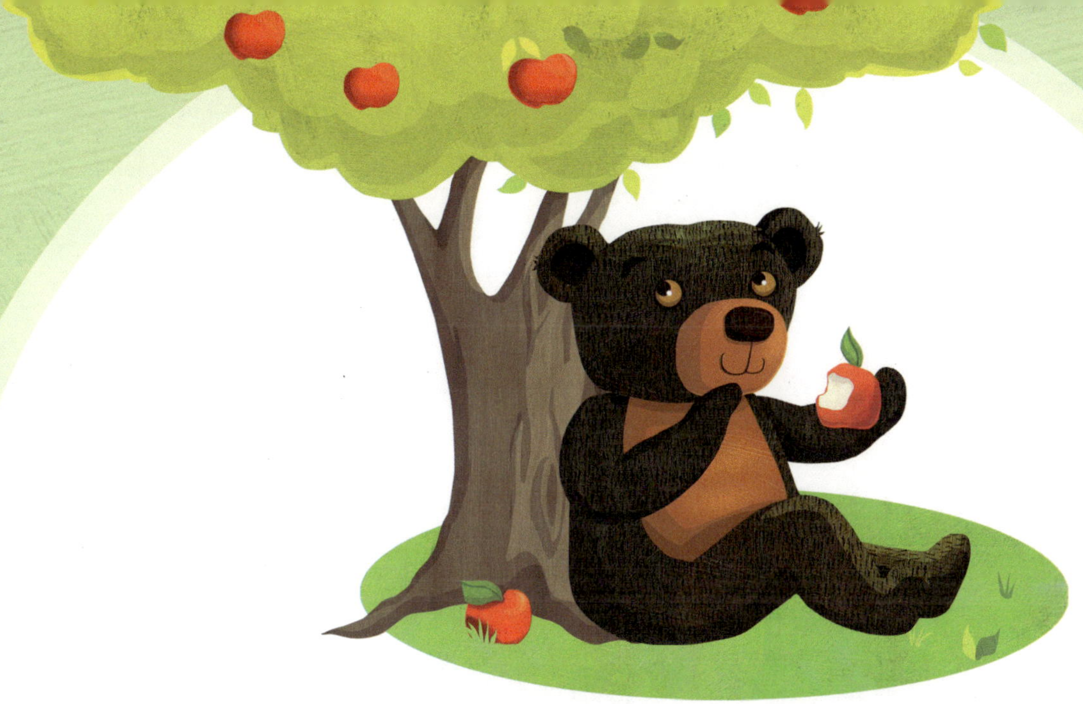

Hey, Boots the Bear, what do you eat?

A Kid's Guide to Fruits and Vegetables

By Beth Dunlap

Registered Dietitian Nutritionist

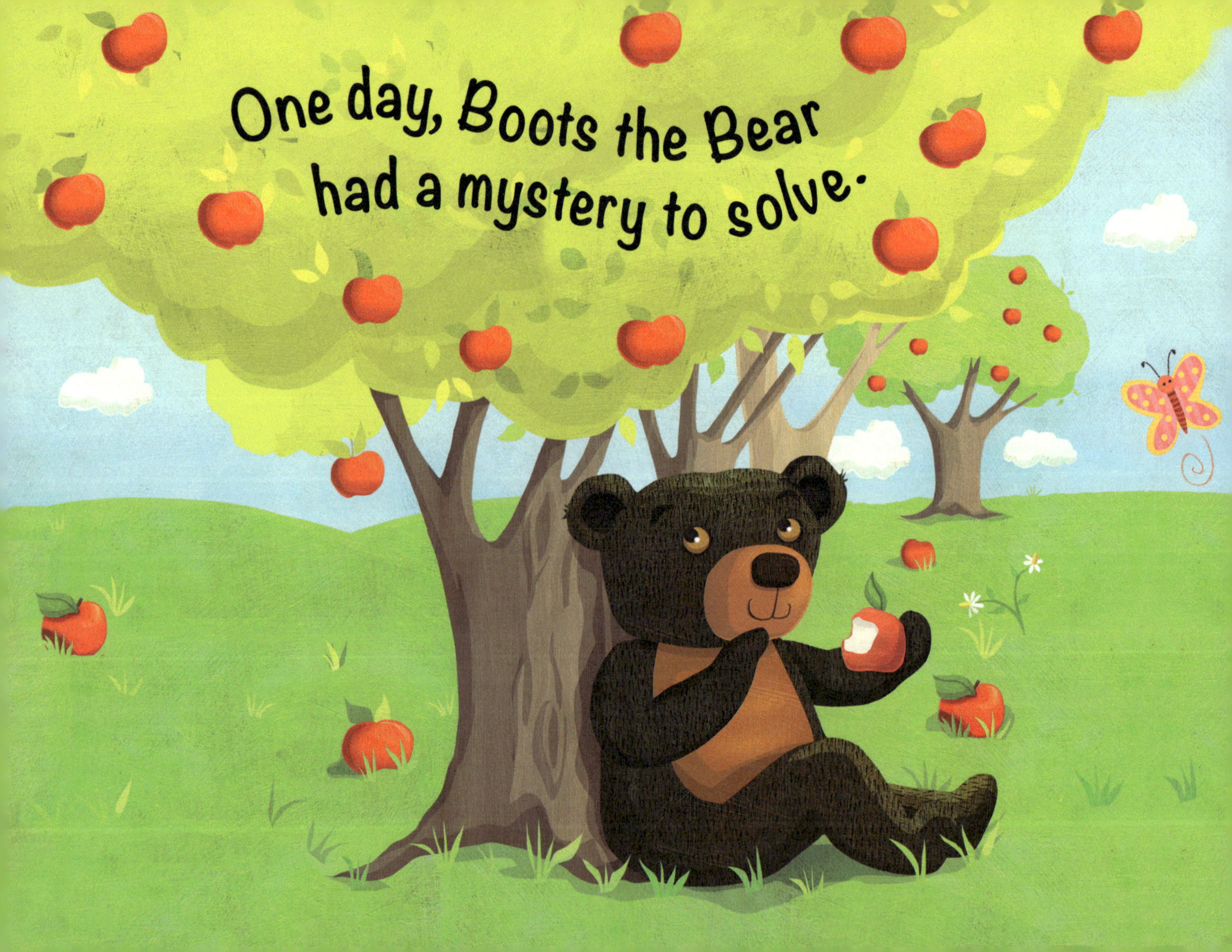

One day, Boots the Bear
had a mystery to solve.

"How do fruits and veggies help me grow, run, and play?" Boots wondered.

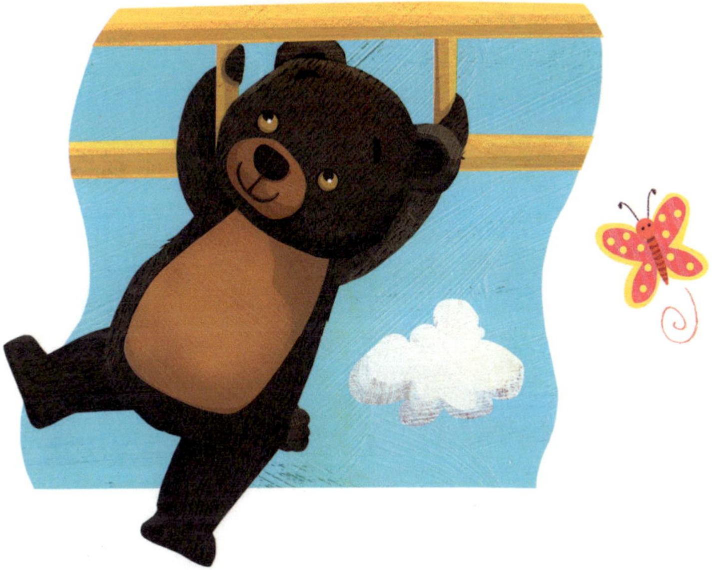

Boots set off to find the answers.

Boots' first stop was to visit Farmer Ward.

Pepper the Puppy was there,
helping in the garden.

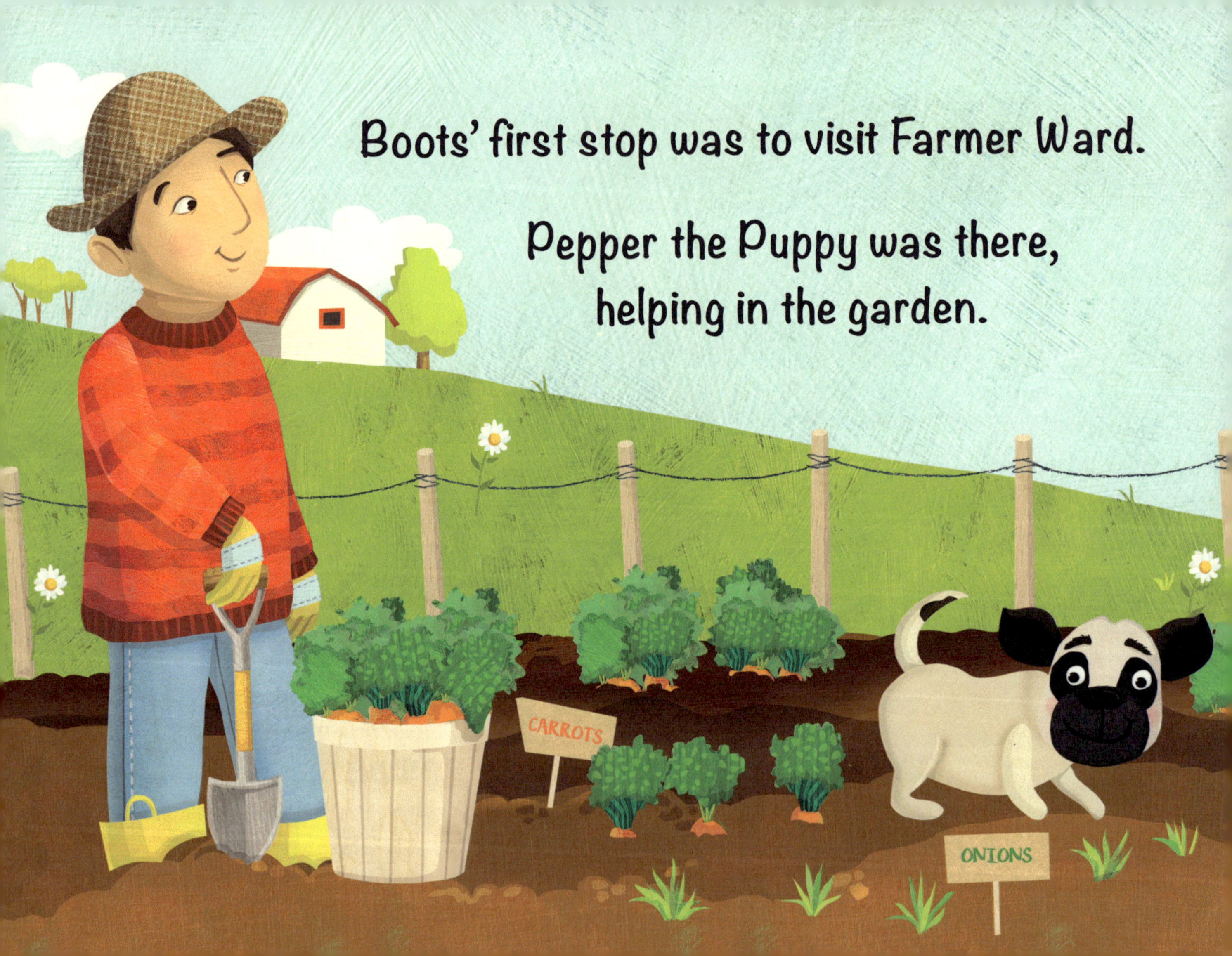

“How do fruits and
veggies help me grow,
run, and play?”
Boots asked.

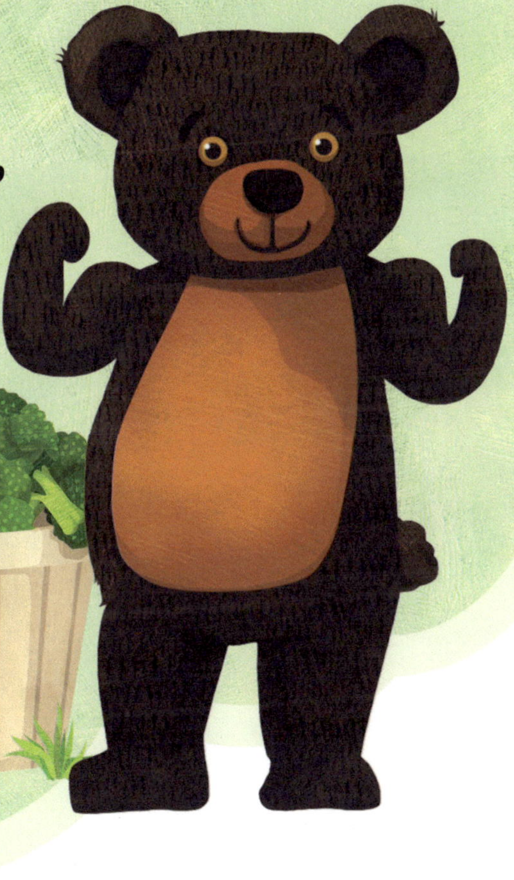

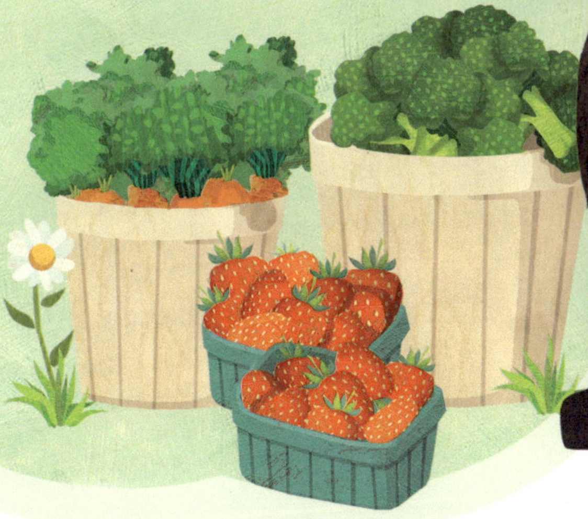

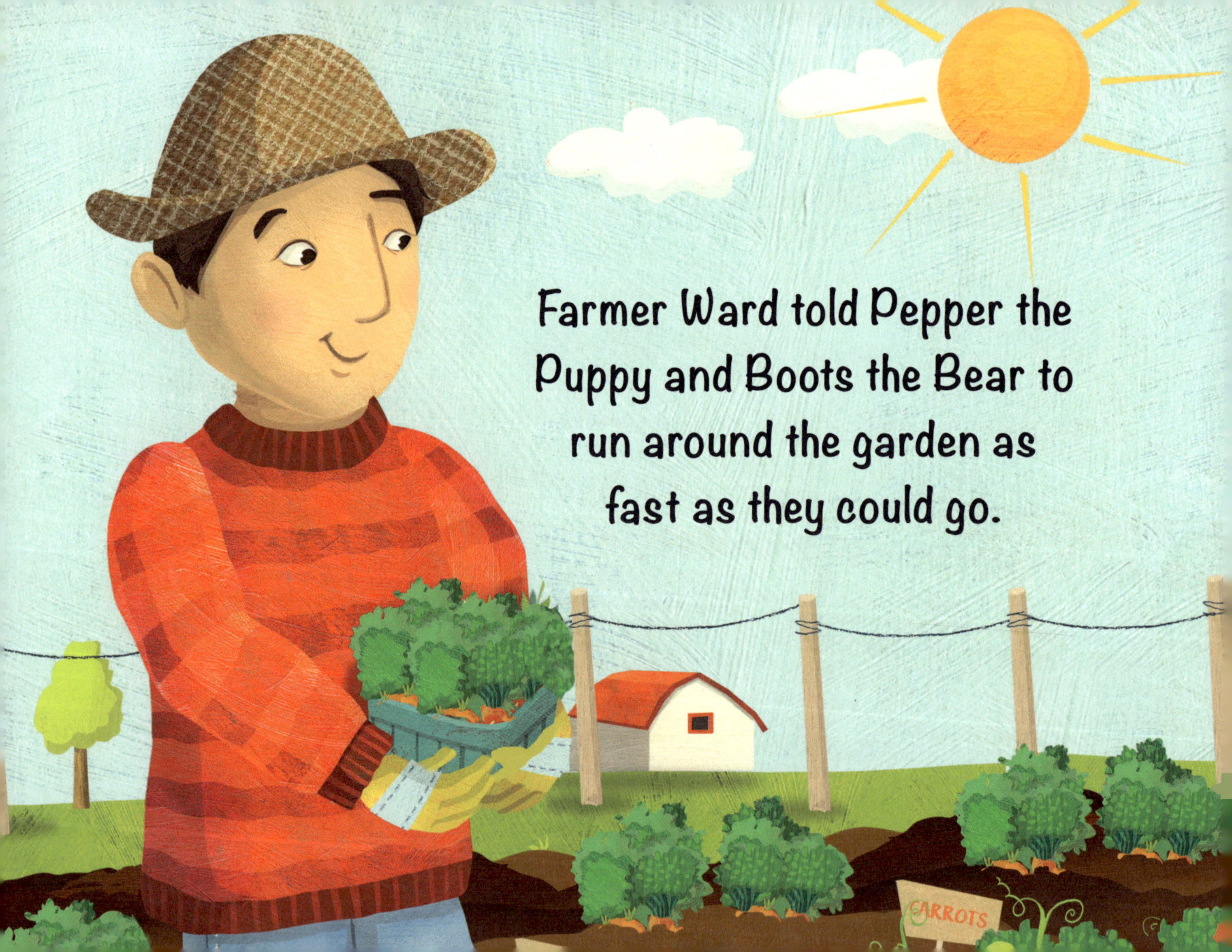

Farmer Ward told Pepper the Puppy and Boots the Bear to run around the garden as fast as they could go.

"Wow, that was fast!"
said Farmer Ward.

Fruits and veggies help give you
energy to run speedy quick.

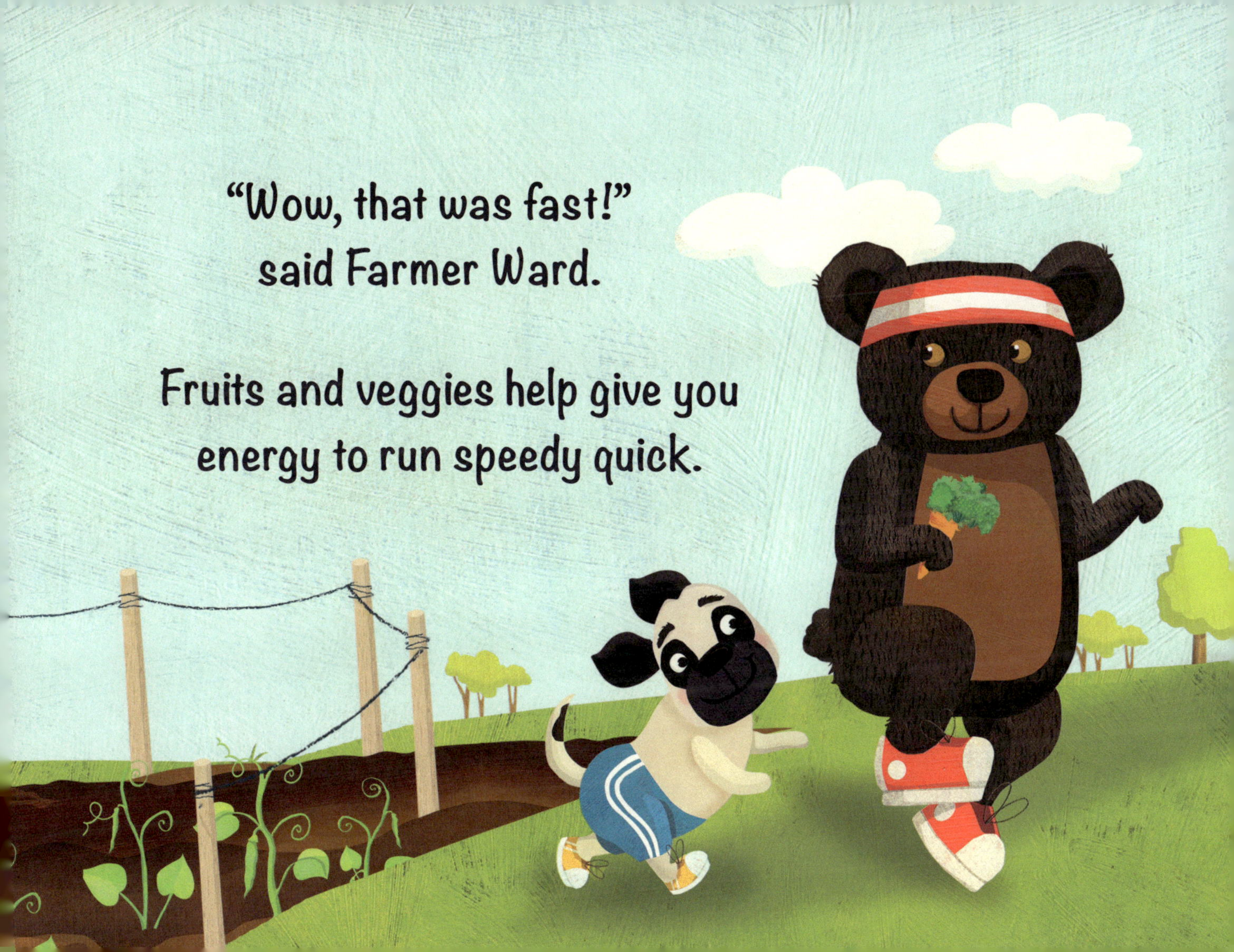

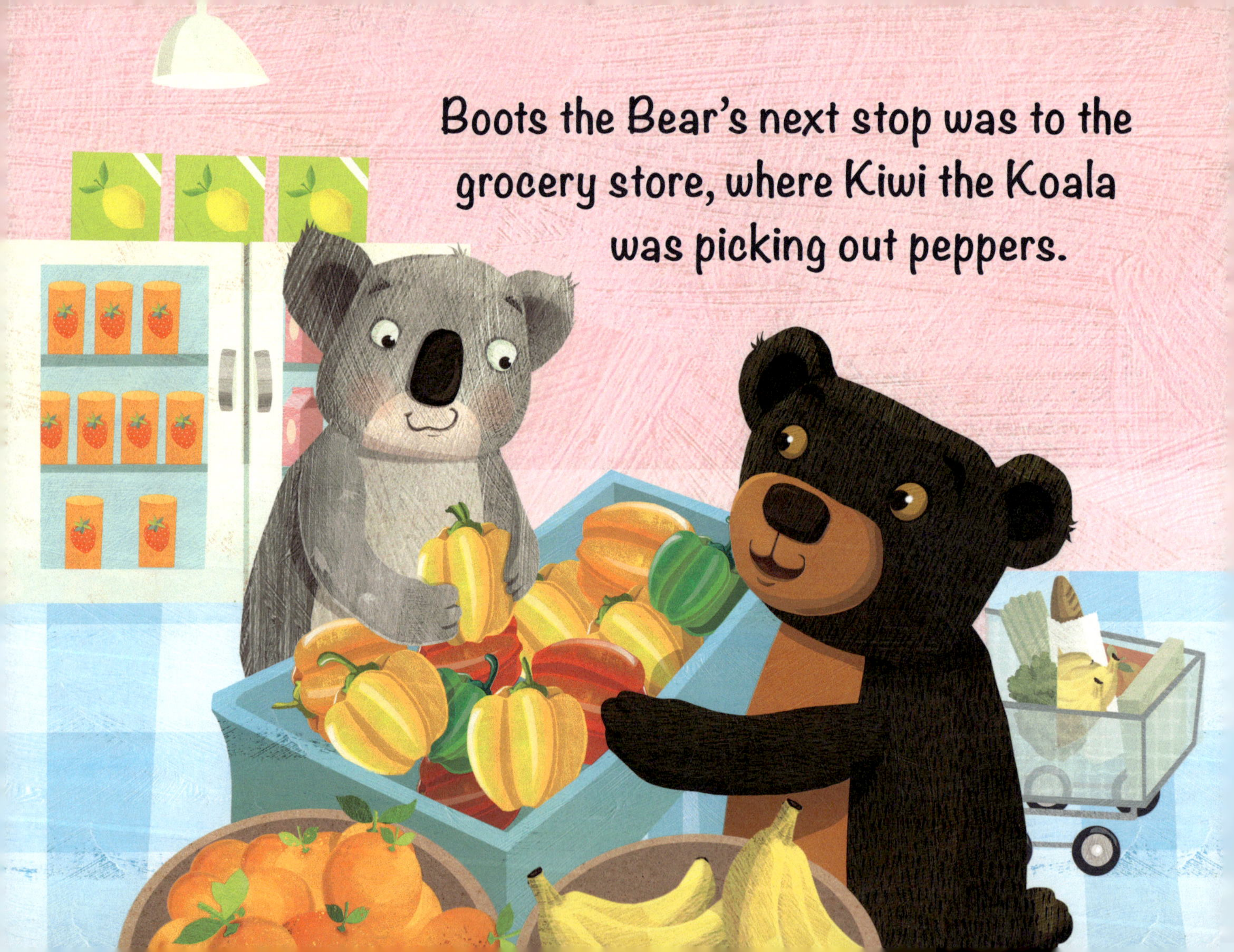

Boots the Bear's next stop was to the grocery store, where Kiwi the Koala was picking out peppers.

"How do fruits and veggies help me grow, run, and play?" Boots asks Kiwi the Koala.

Kiwi replied, "Fruits and veggies help with super sight and healthy bones."

The more you eat, the more you grow!

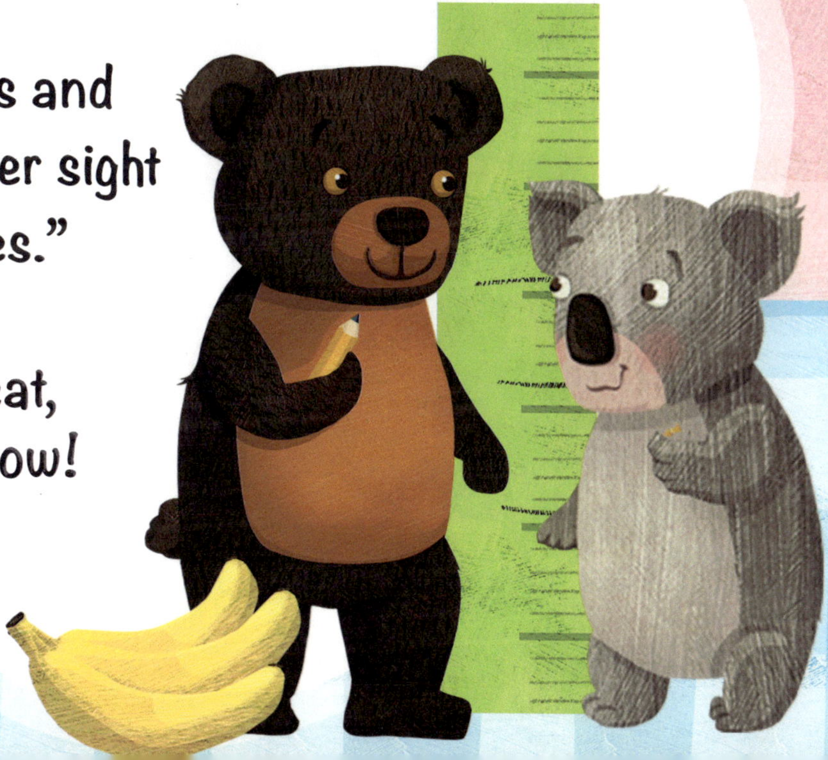

Next, Boots the Bear met Beau the Bunny at the Farmer's Market to buy some strawberries.

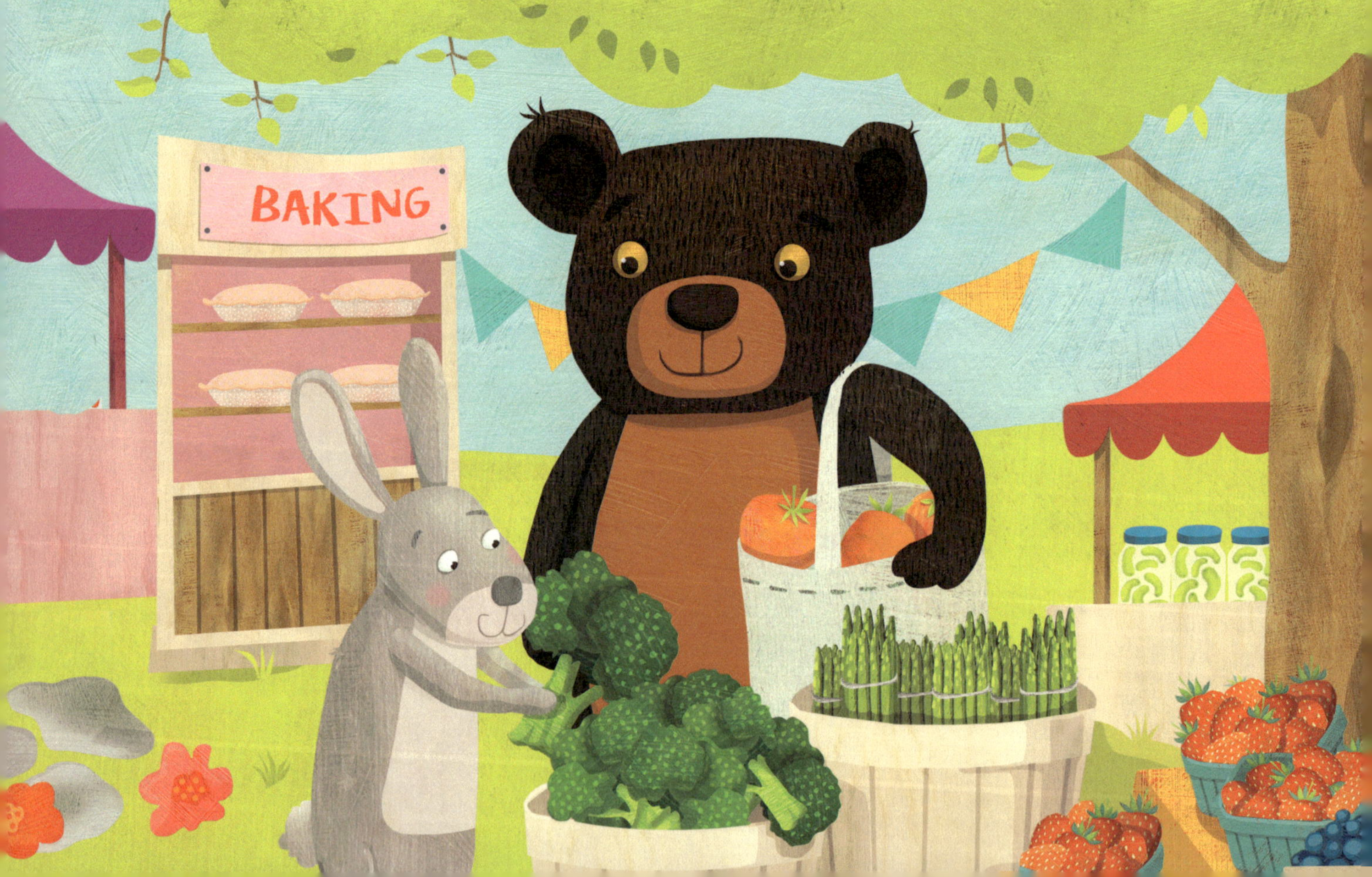

"How do fruits and veggies help me grow, run, and play?" Boots asks Beau.

Beau tells Boots to try to blink his eyes, smile really big, and give his arm a tap-tap-tap to feel his strong bones.

Beau says, "Fruits and veggies help your body move and play, from the tip of your head all the way to your toes."

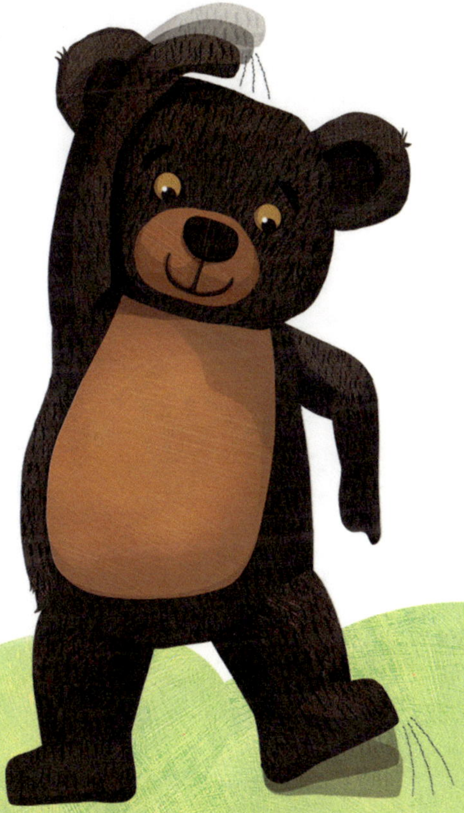

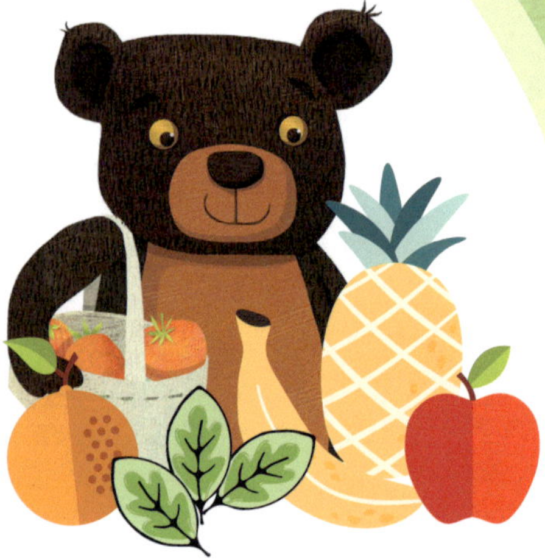

How do fruits and veggies help Boots the Bear?

Growth

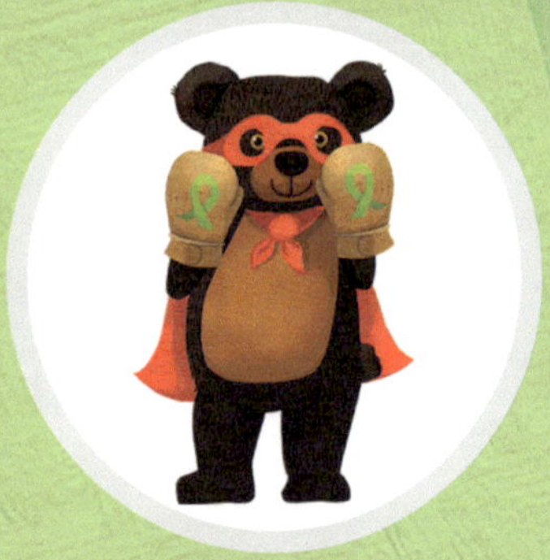

Fight Illness

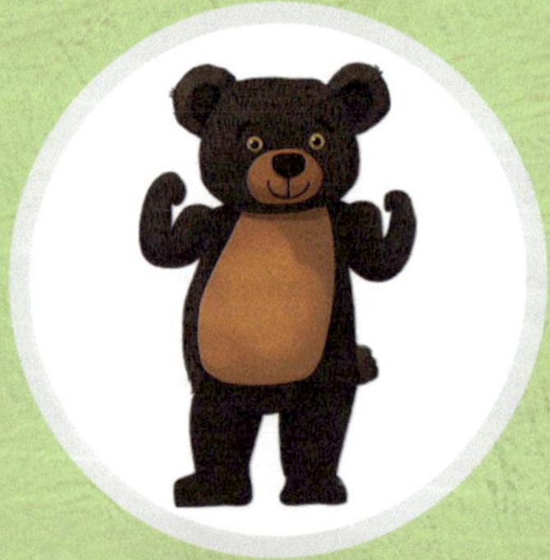

Build Muscles

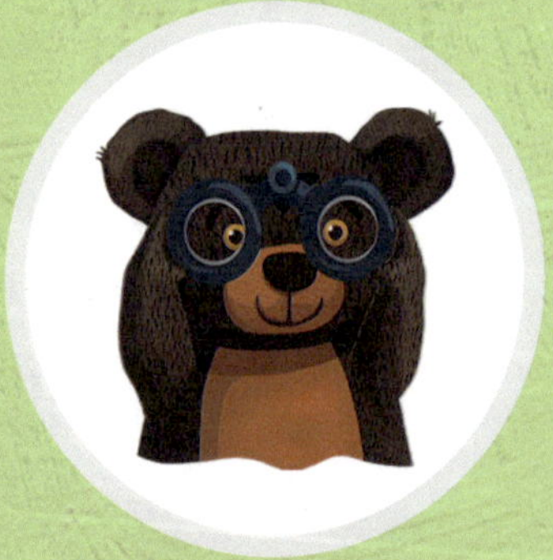

Improve Vision

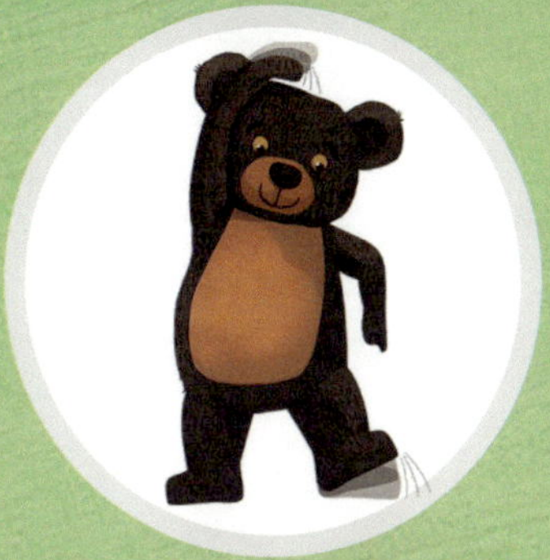

Coordination

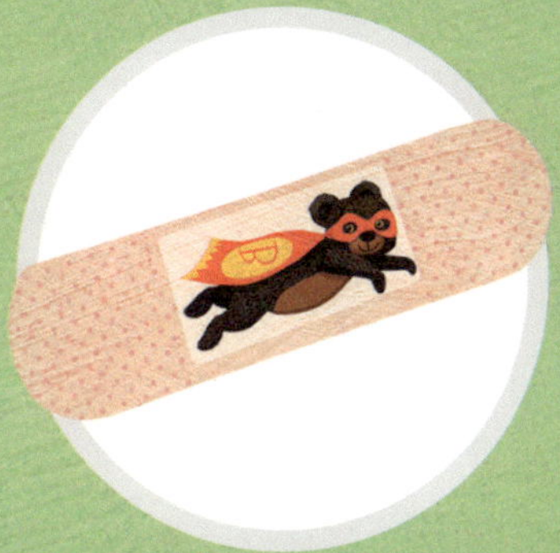

Heal Wounds

Healthy Heart

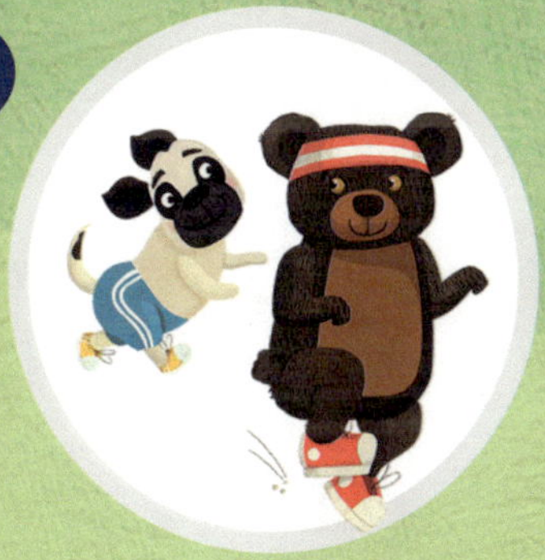

Exercise

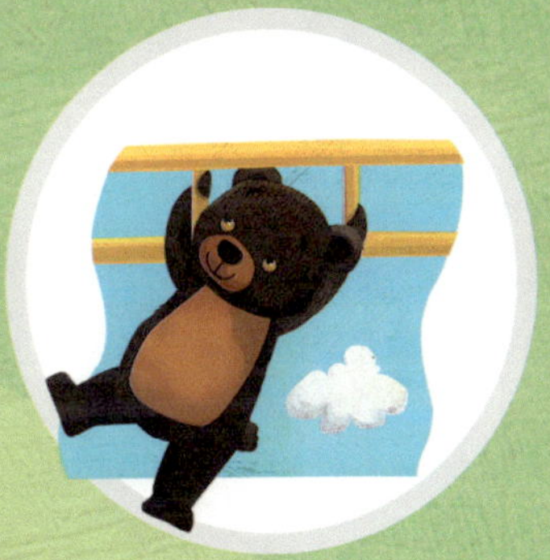

Energy for Play

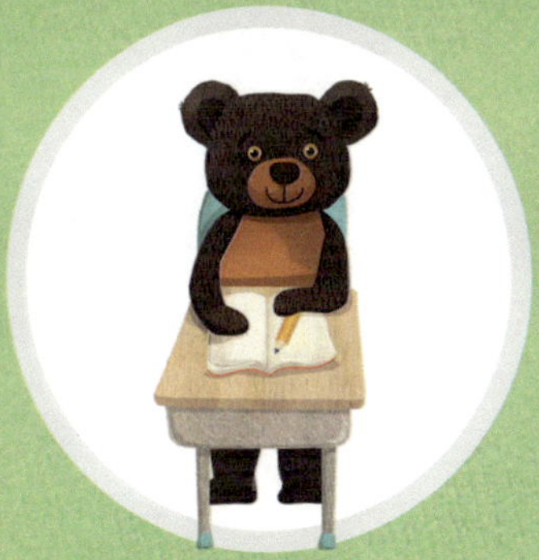

Brain Smart

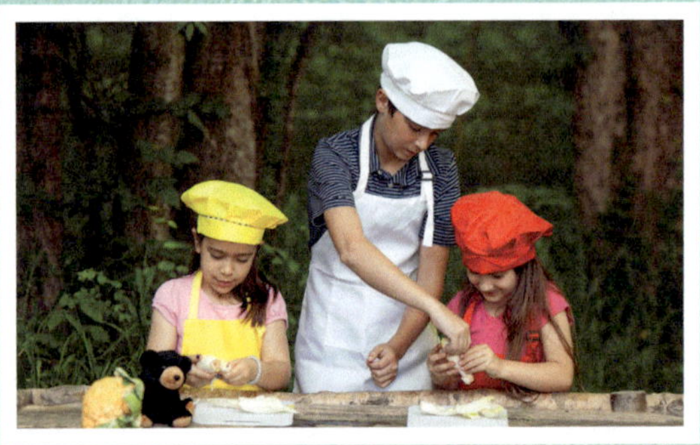
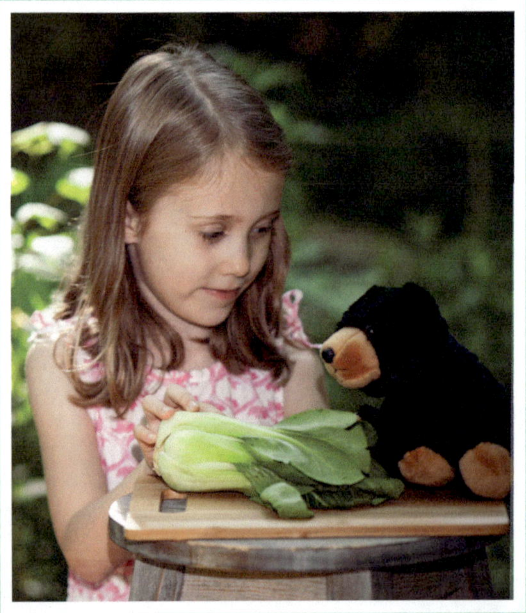
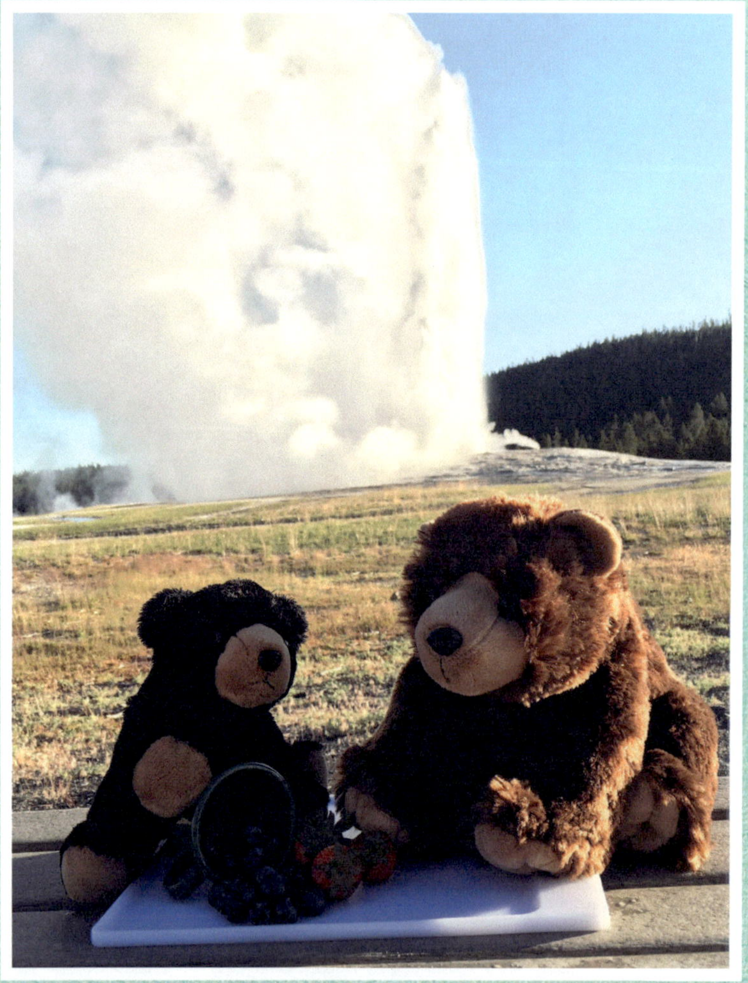

Hey, Boots the Bear, what do you eat to help you grow, run, and play?

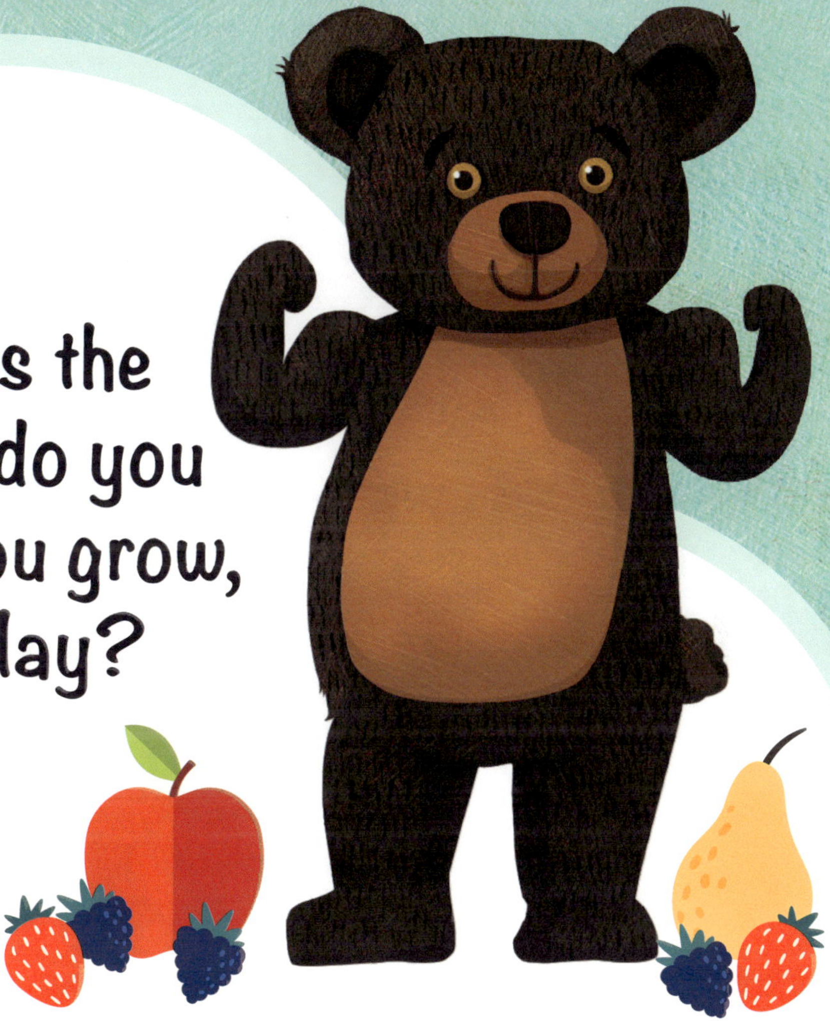

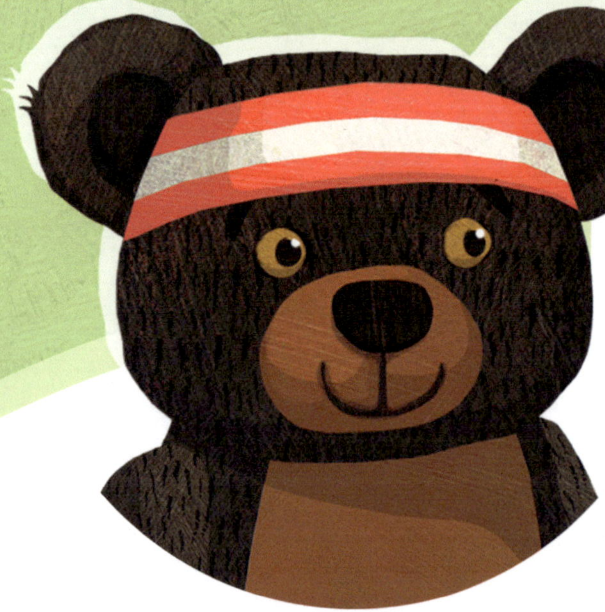

I eat an 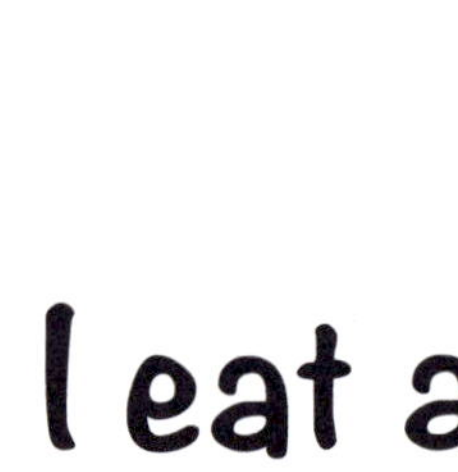

APPLE

to help me hike
to the peak.

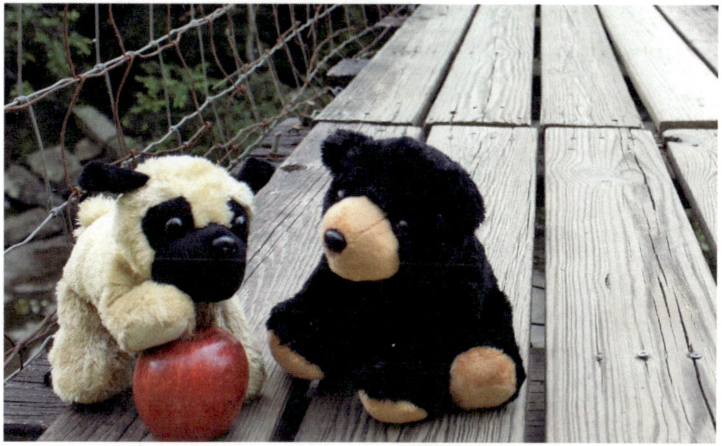

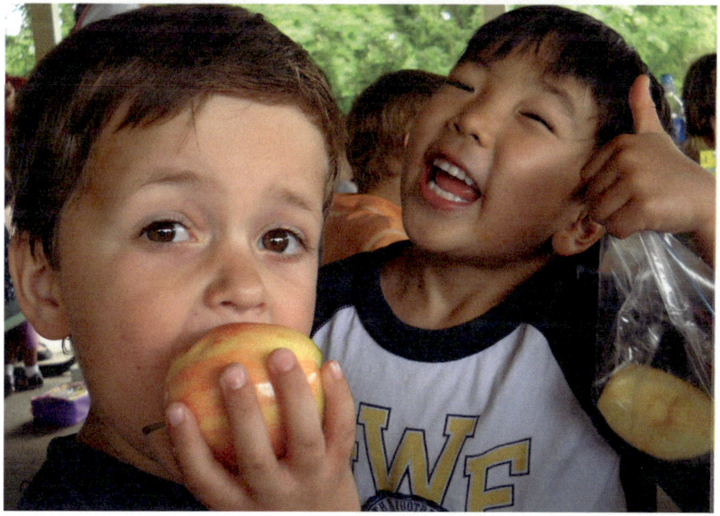

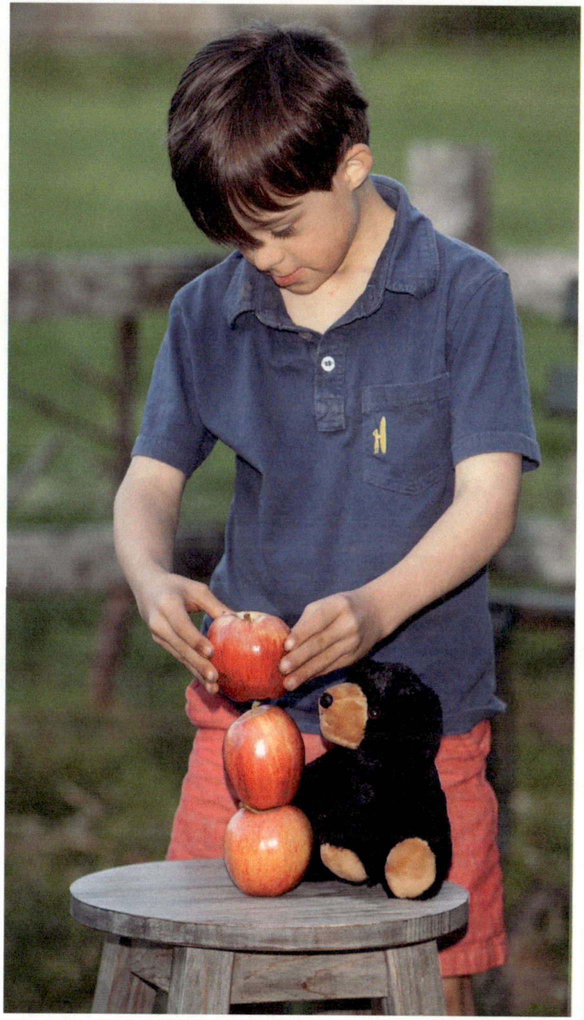

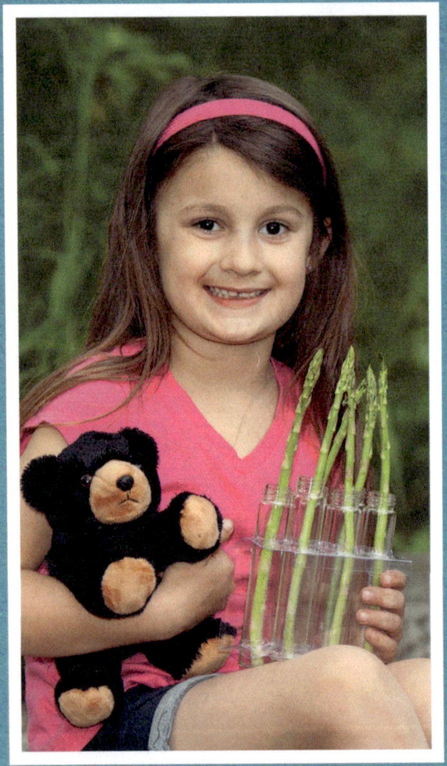

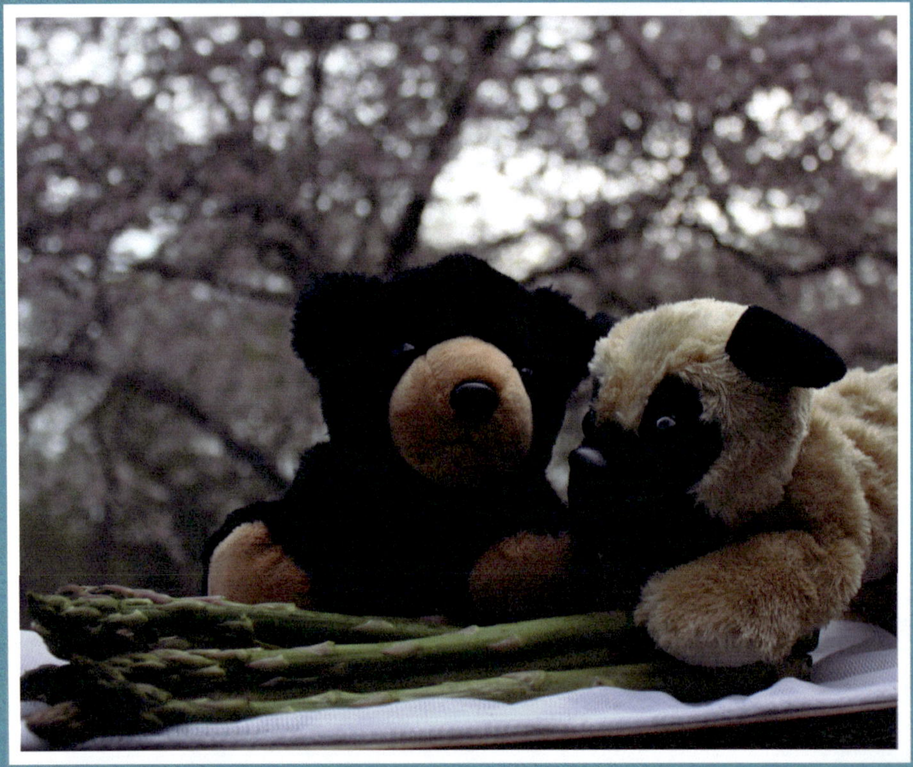

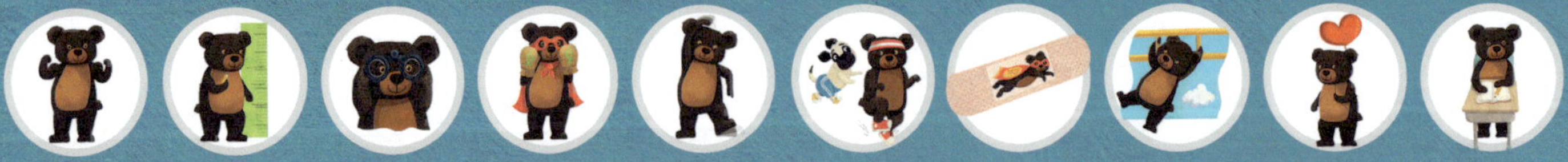

I eat
ASPARAGUS
to help my tummy
feel tip-top.

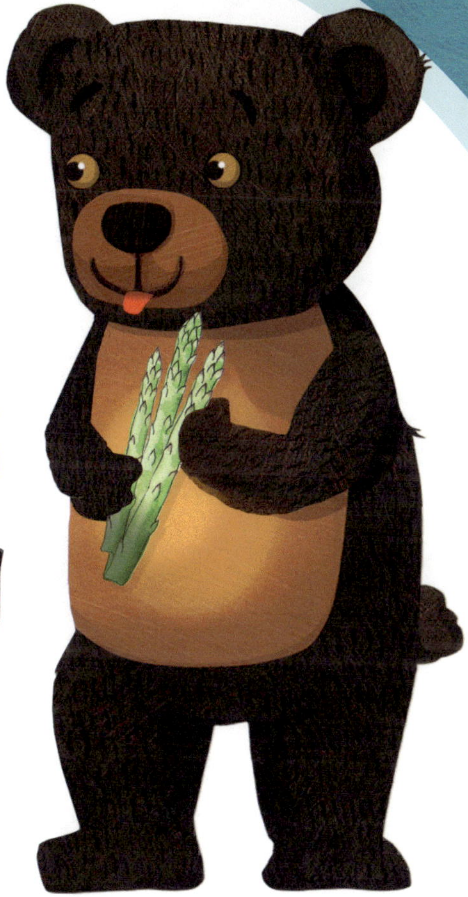

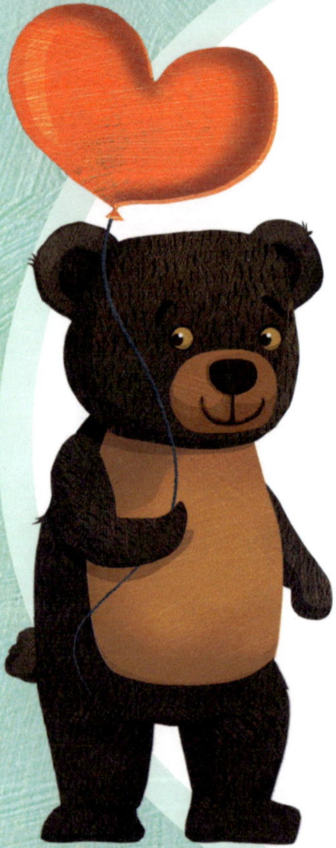

I eat an 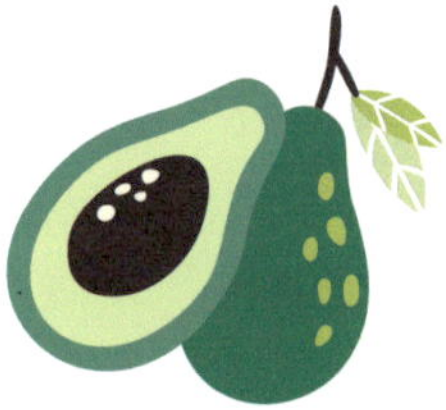

AVOCADO

to help my heart
beat ❤ beat ❤ beat.

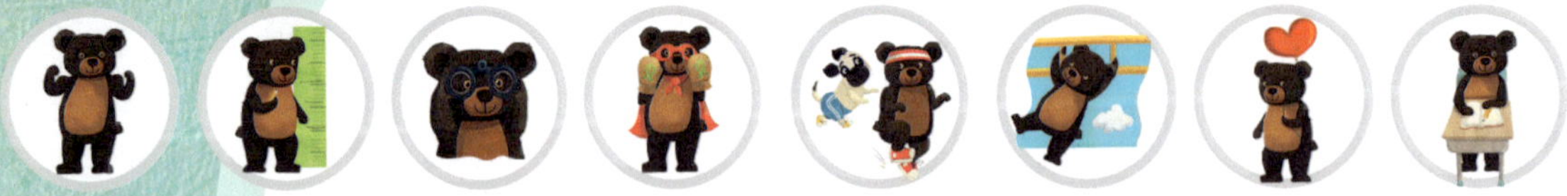

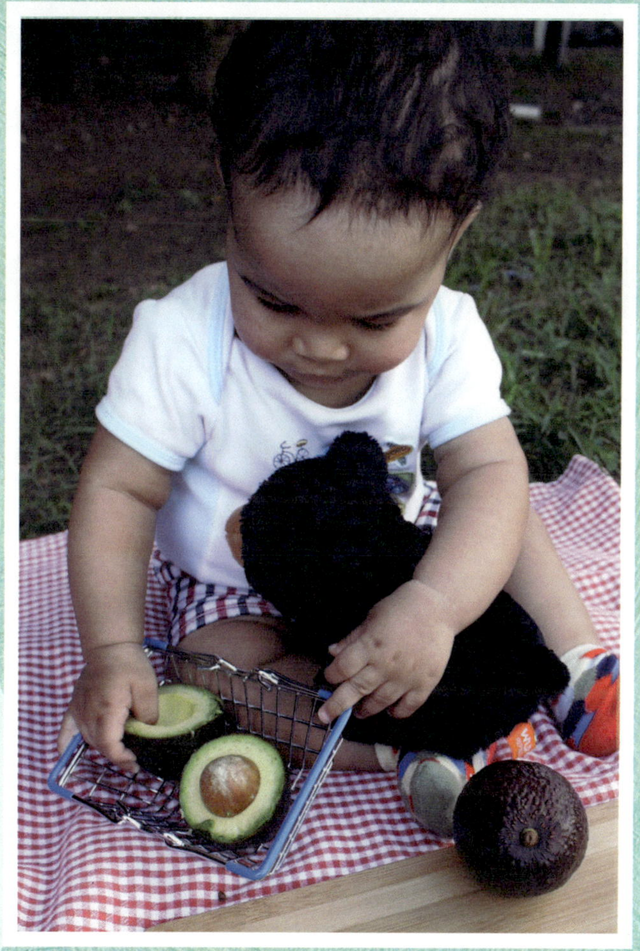

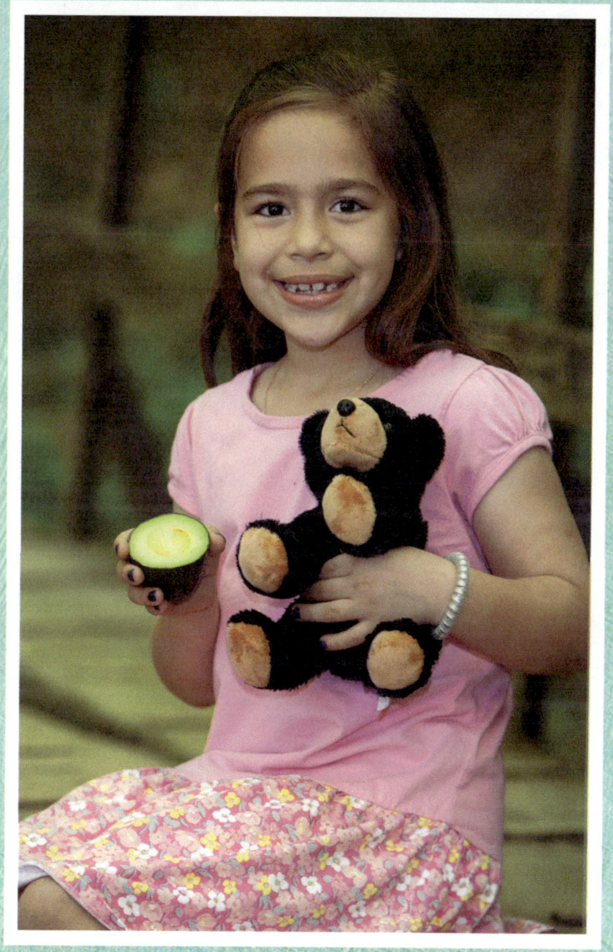

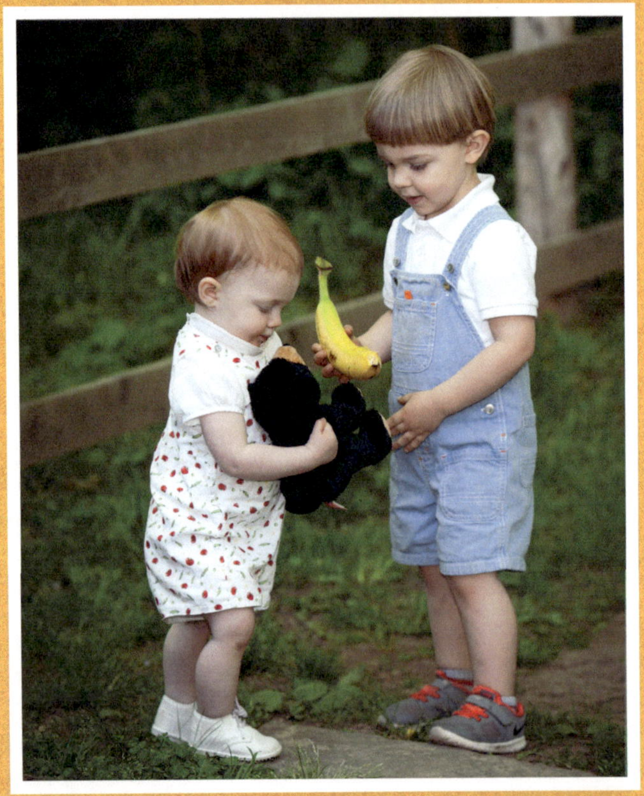

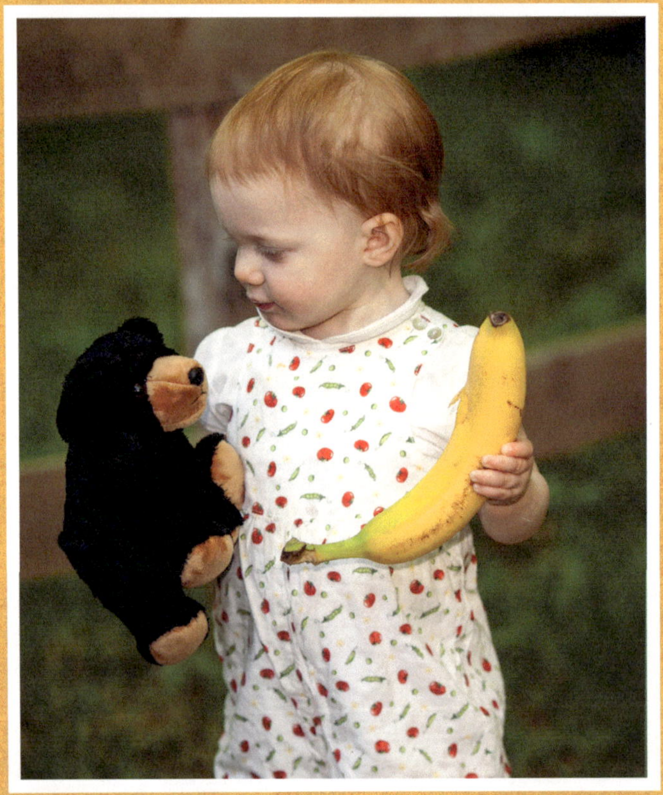

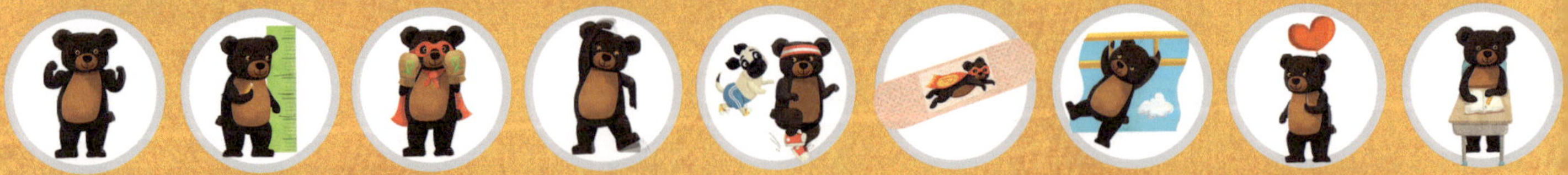

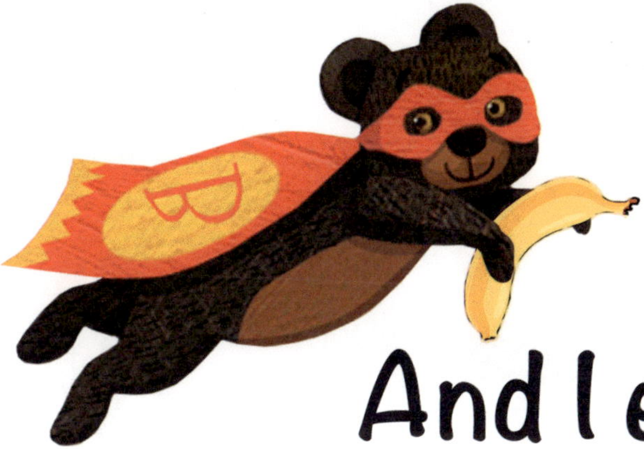

And I eat

BANANAS

to help me blast
around super-fast.

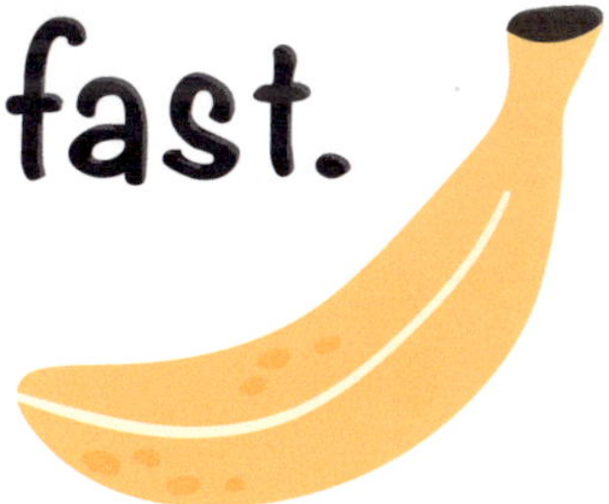

Hey, Boots the Bear,
what do you eat?

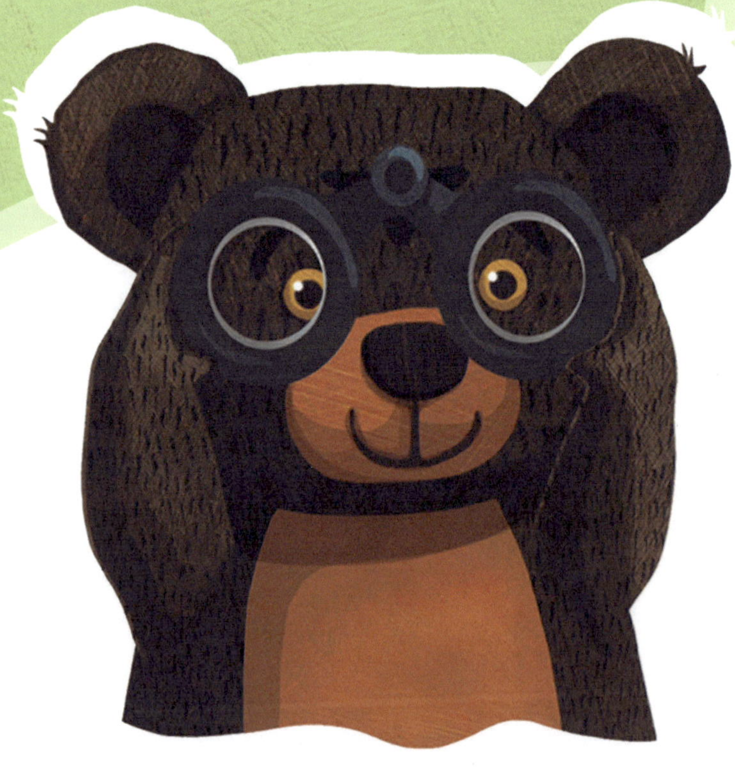

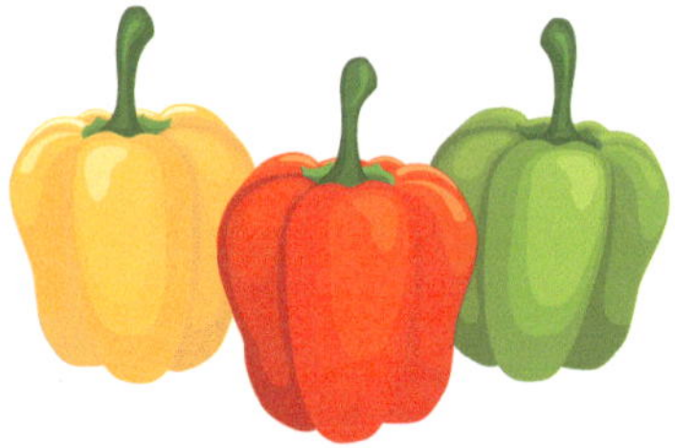

I eat

BELL PEPPERS

to help my
super sight.

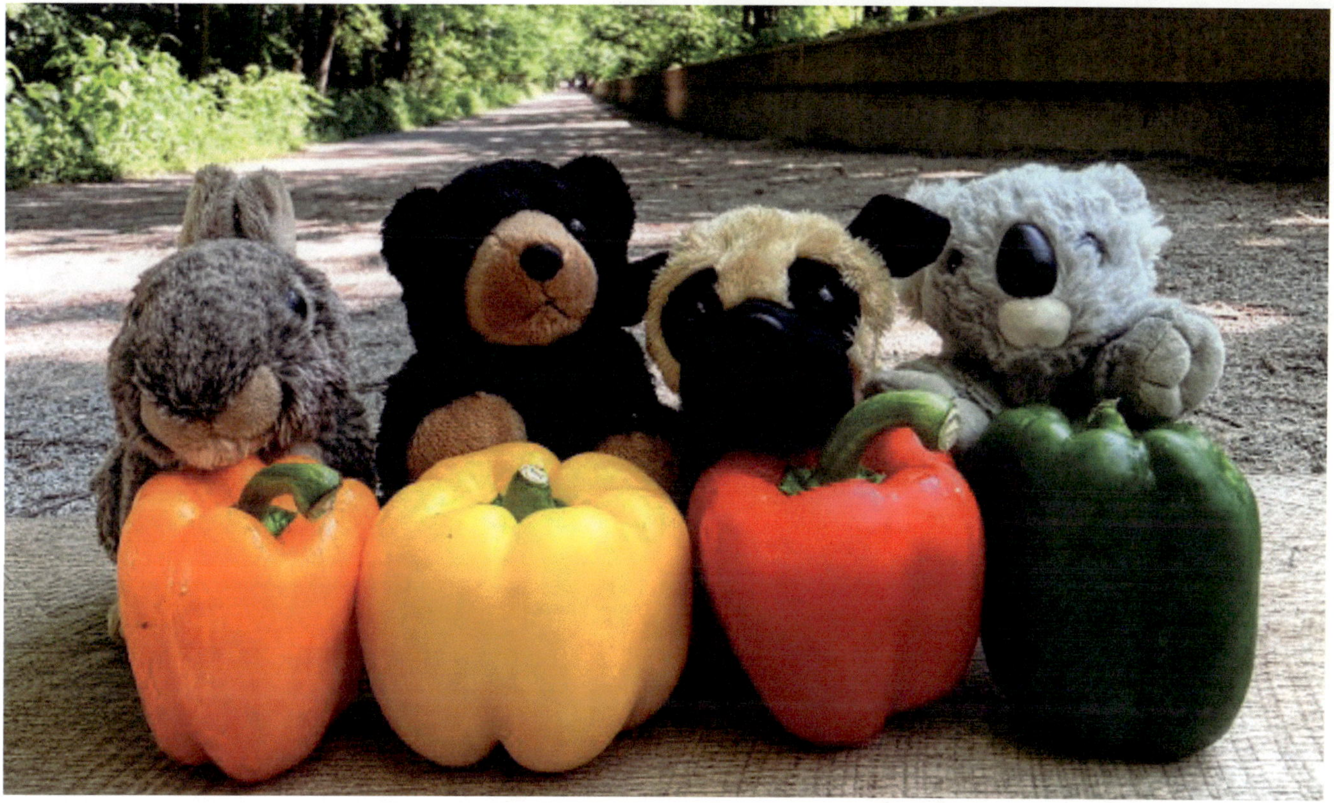

 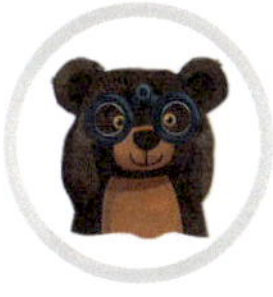   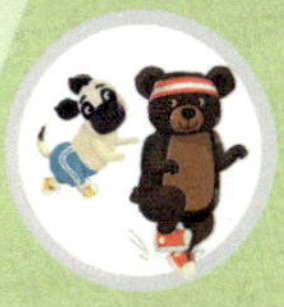 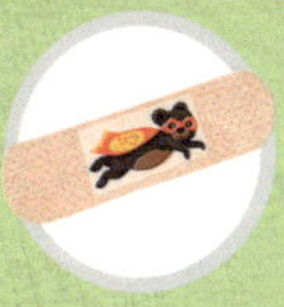   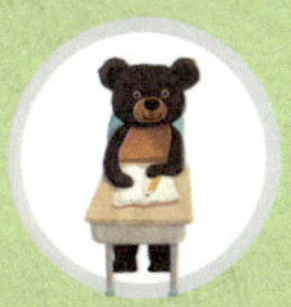

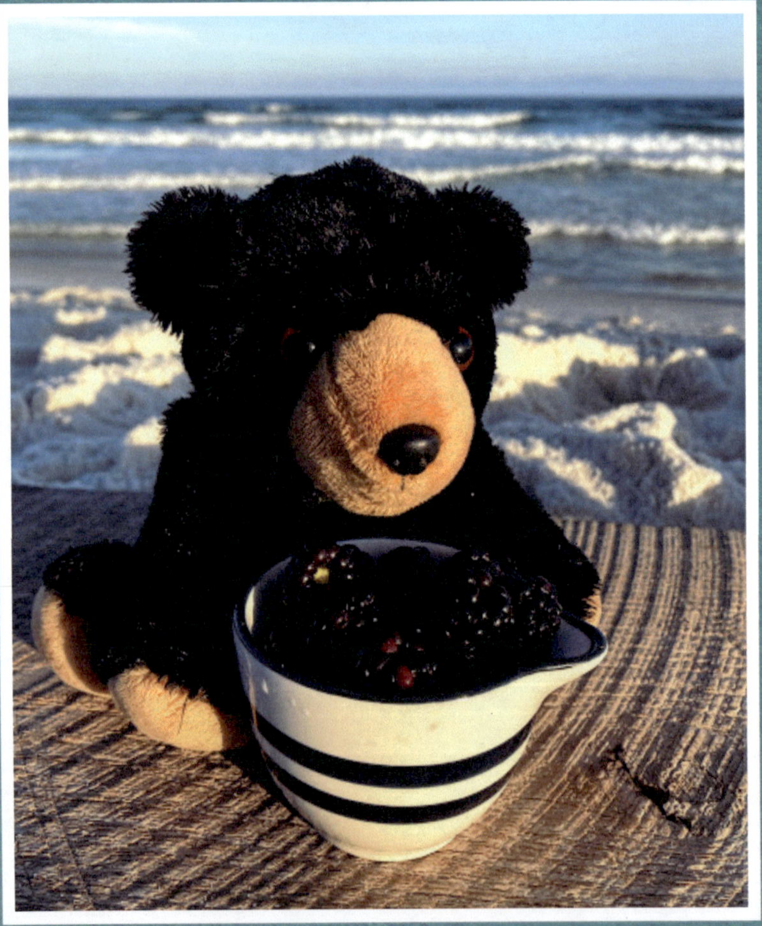

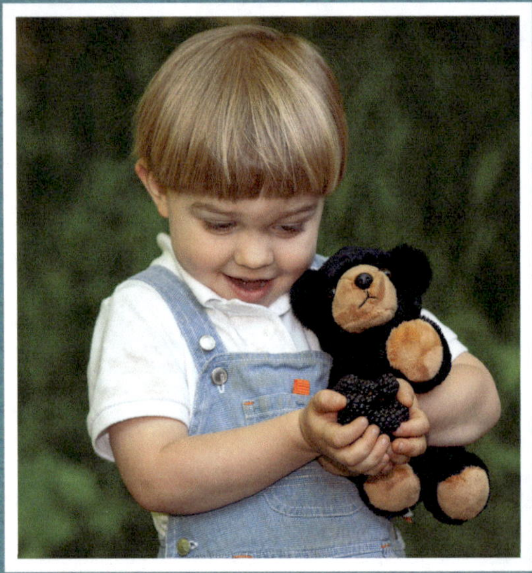

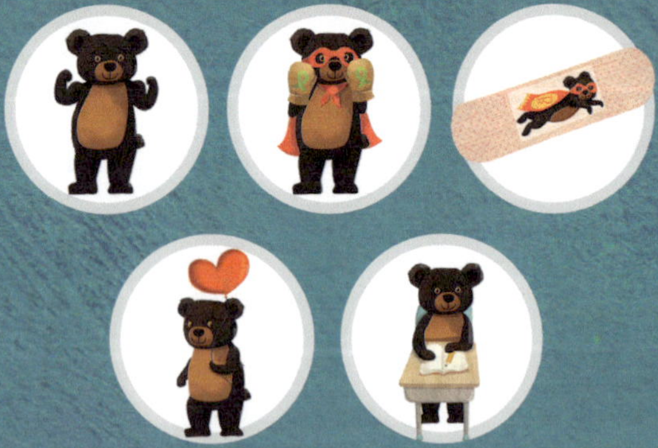

I eat

BLACKBERRIES

to help my legs pedal
fast on family bike rides.

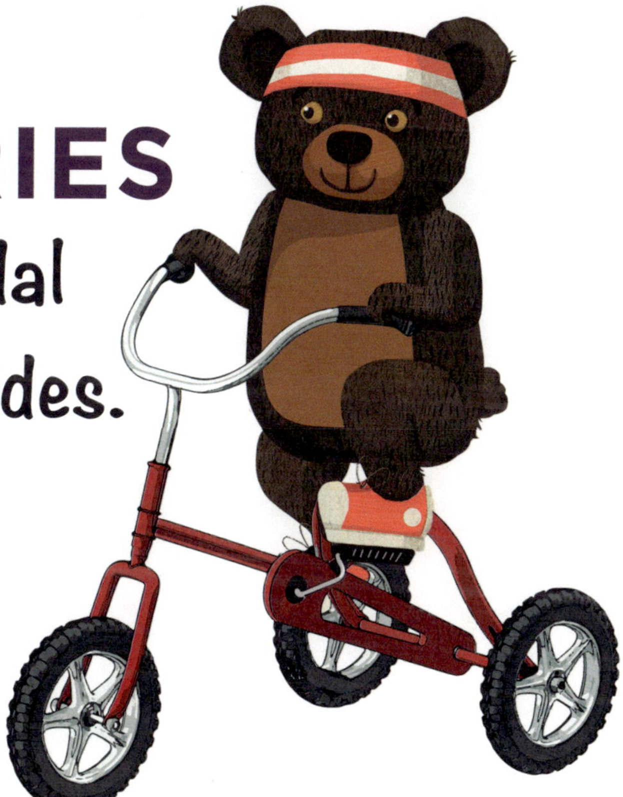

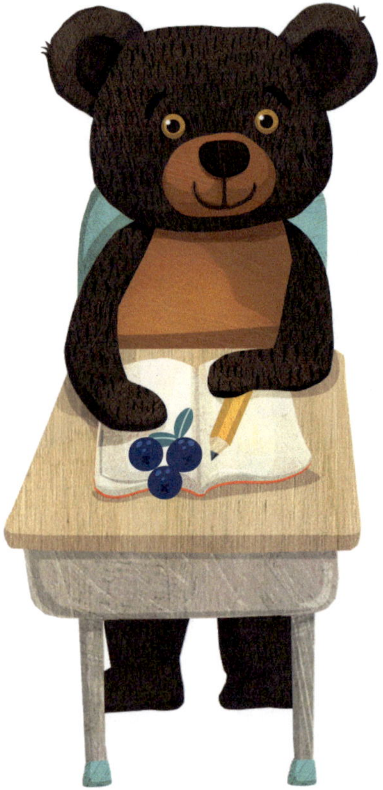

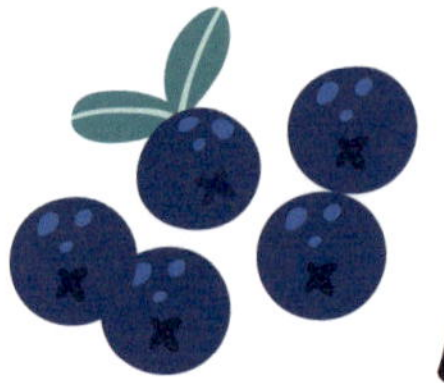

And I eat

BLUEBERRIES

to give me a smart start to the day.

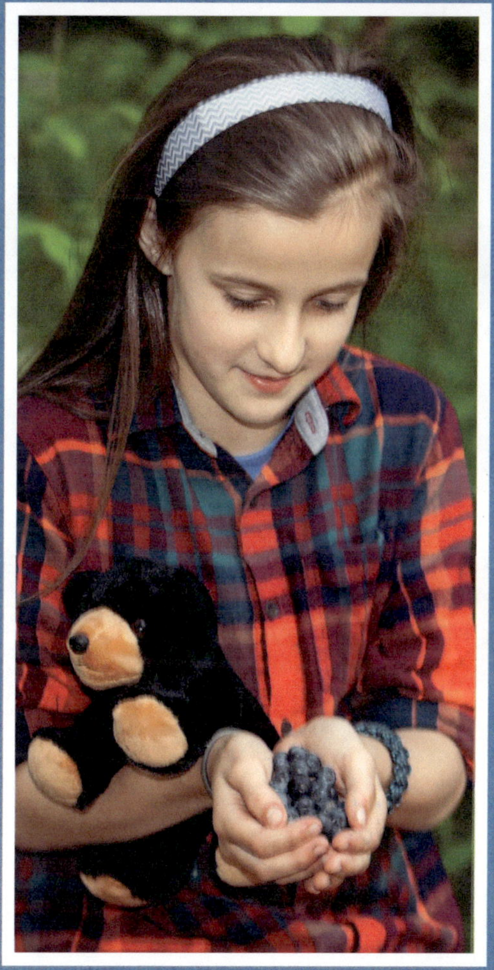

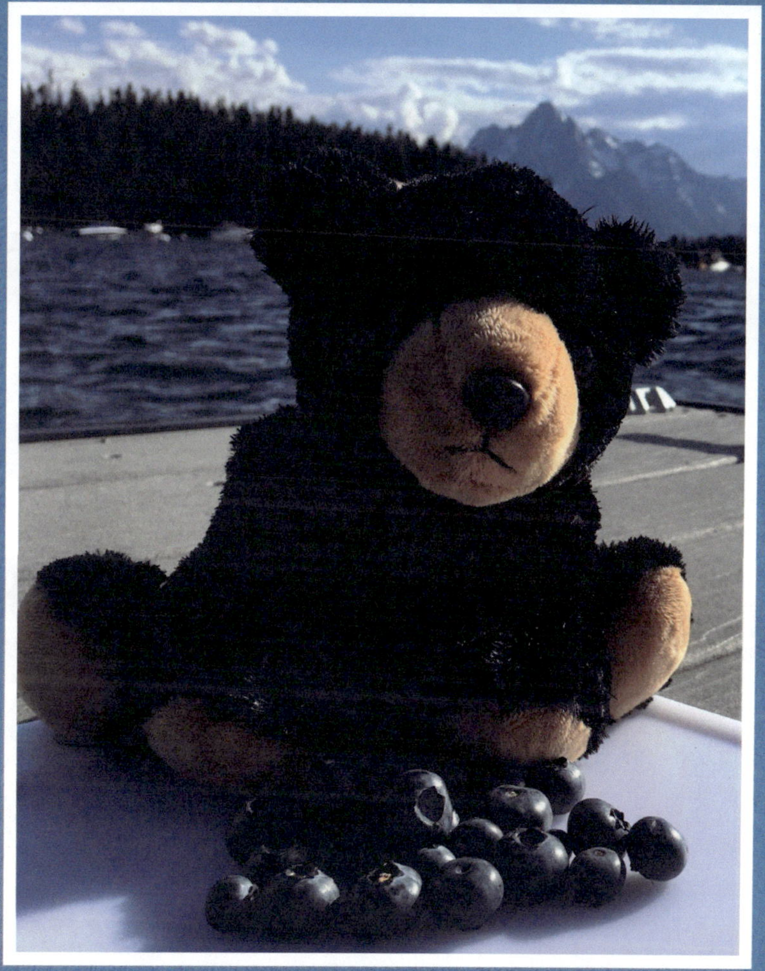

Hey, Boots the Bear, what do your friends eat?

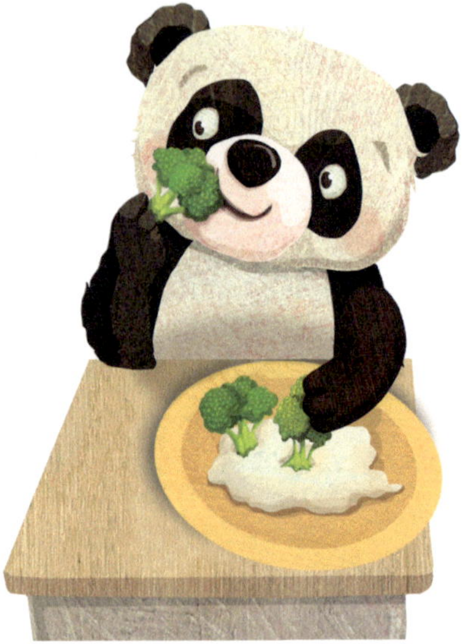

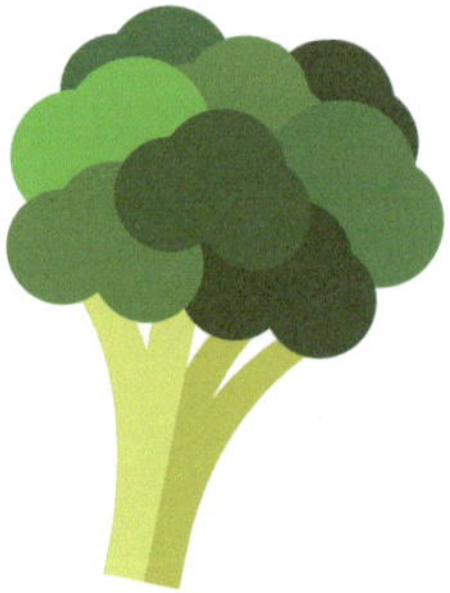

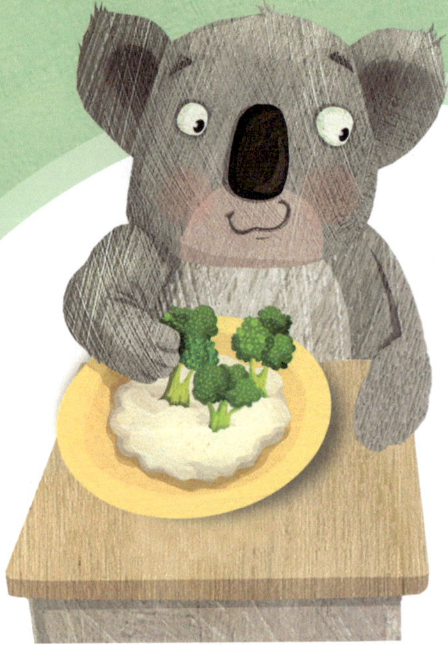

Boots' friends eat

BROCCOLI

to help them be super students at school.

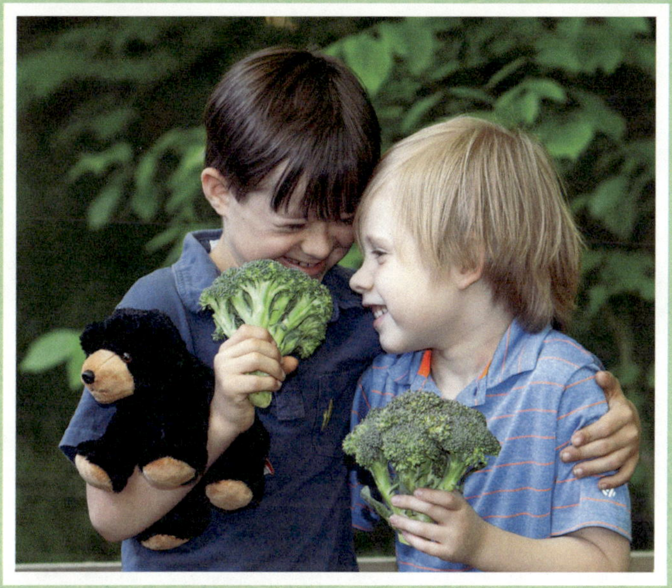
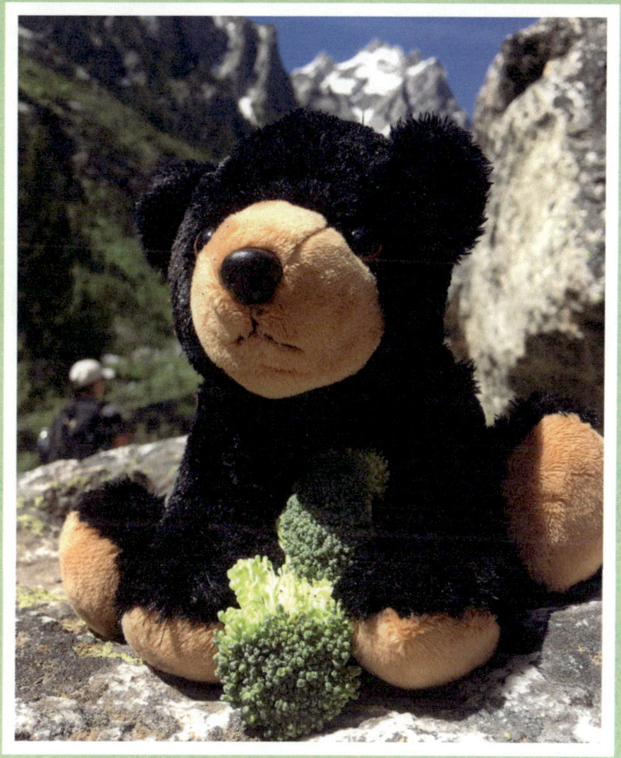

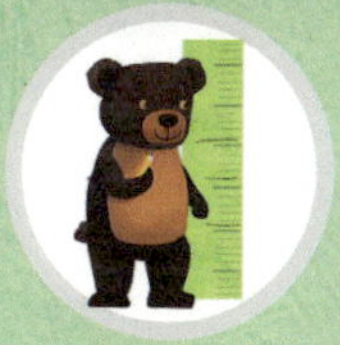
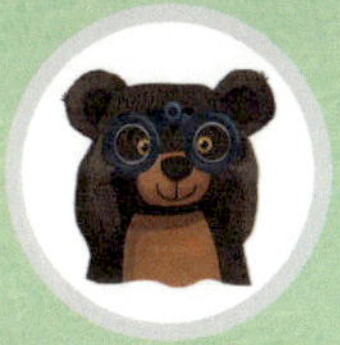

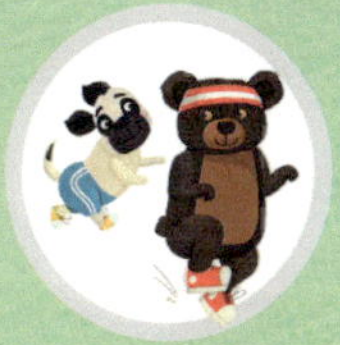
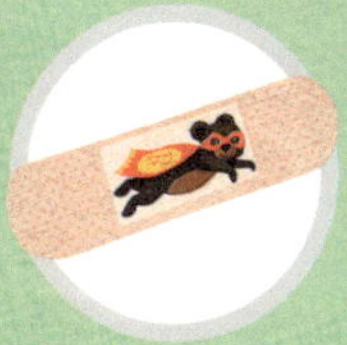

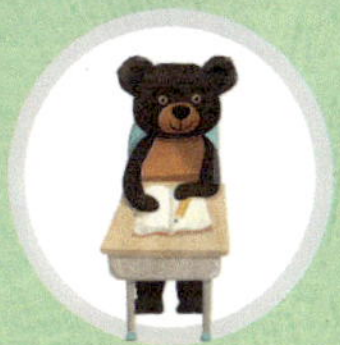

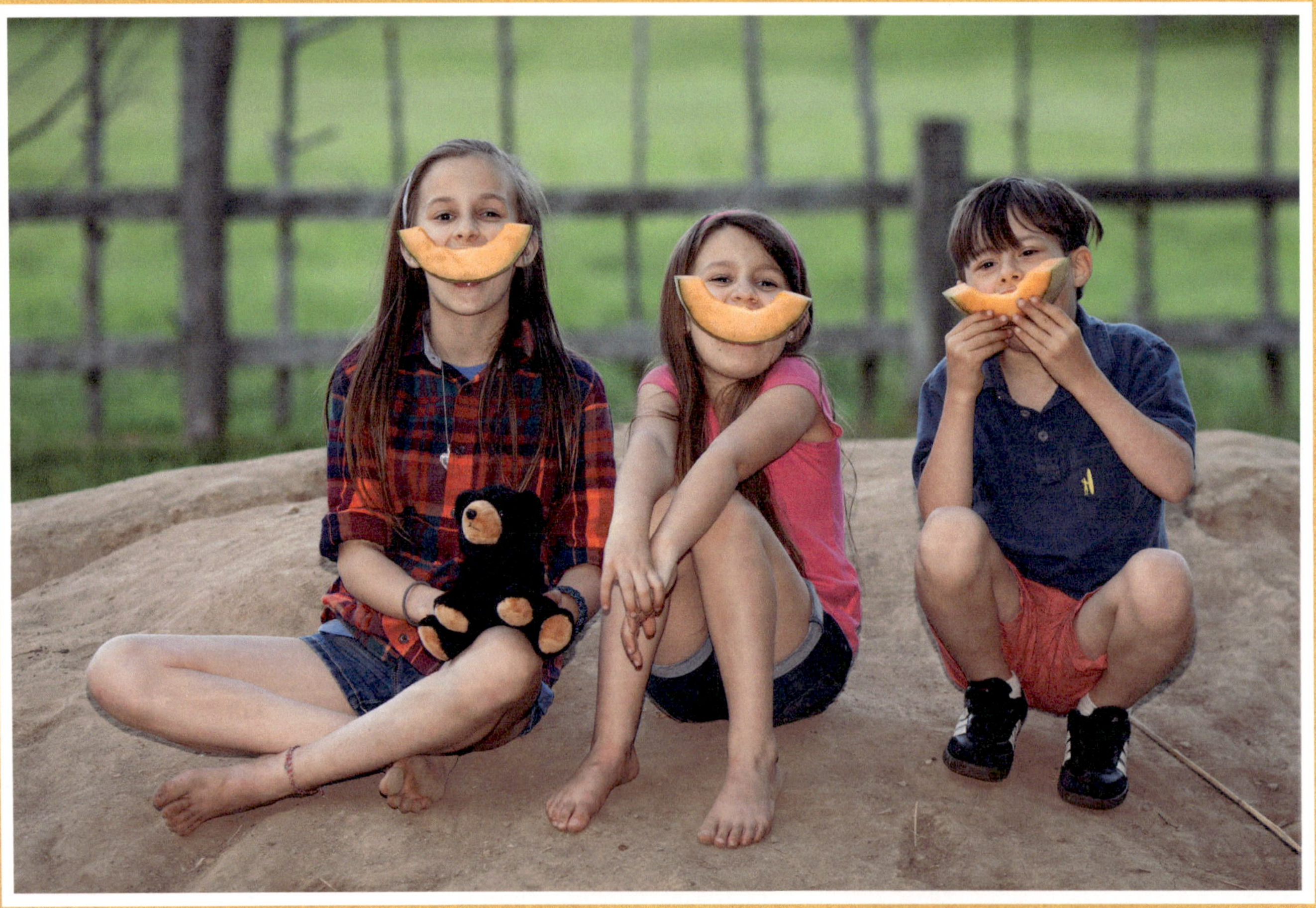

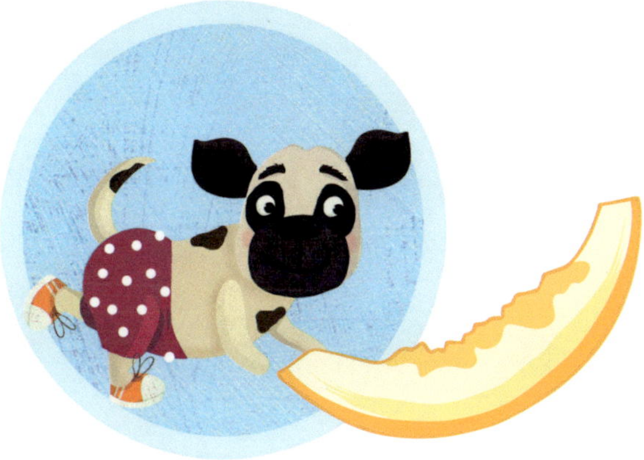

Pepper the Puppy eats

CANTALOUPE

to help him run, jump, hop, and skip.

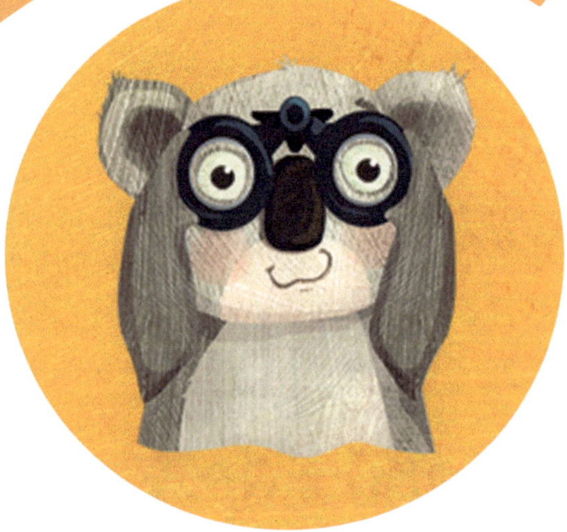

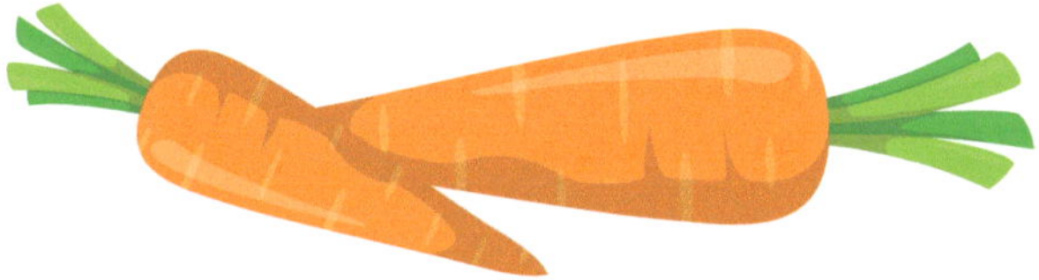

And Kiwi the Koala eats

CARROTS

to help give him X-ray vision.

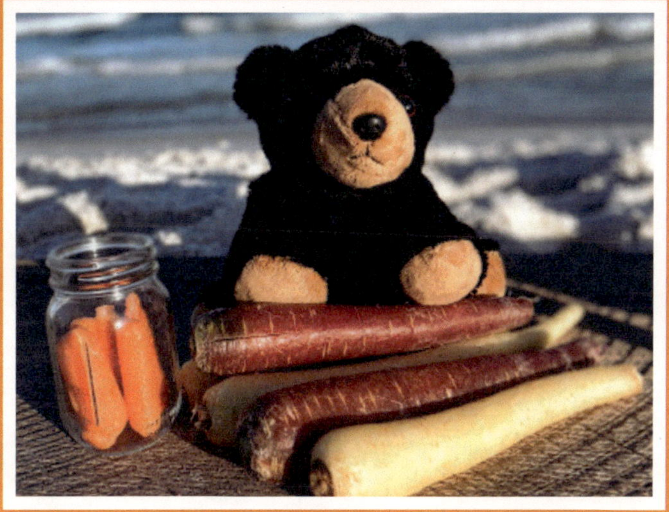
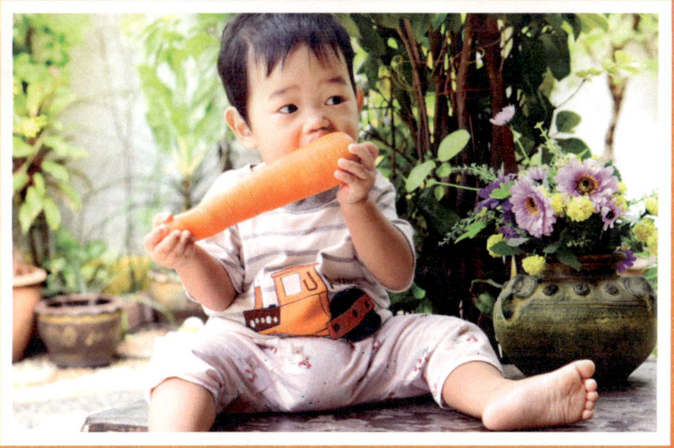
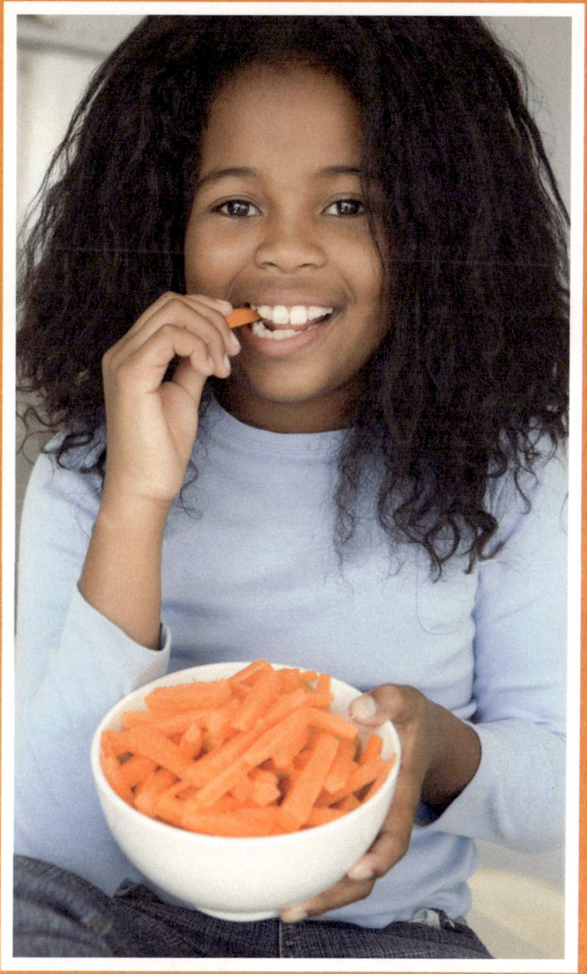

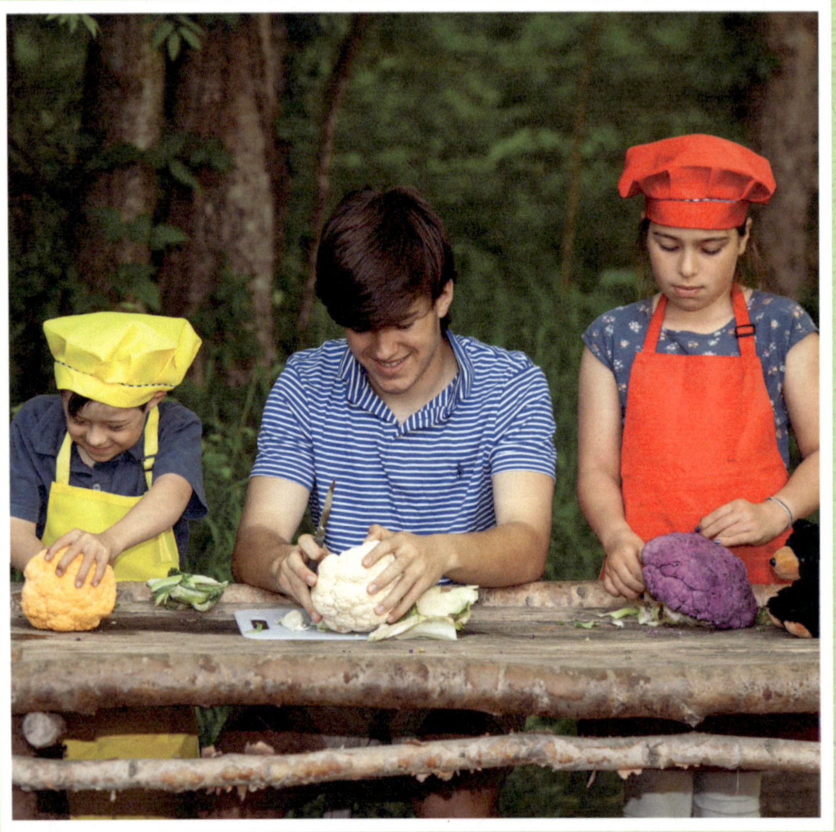
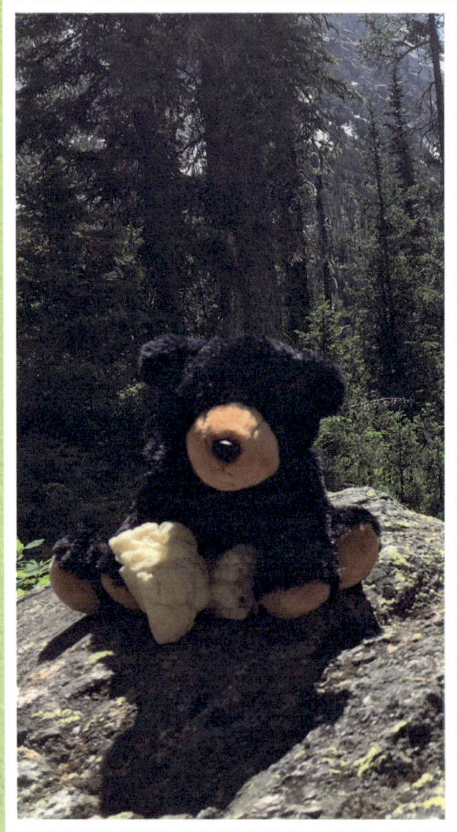
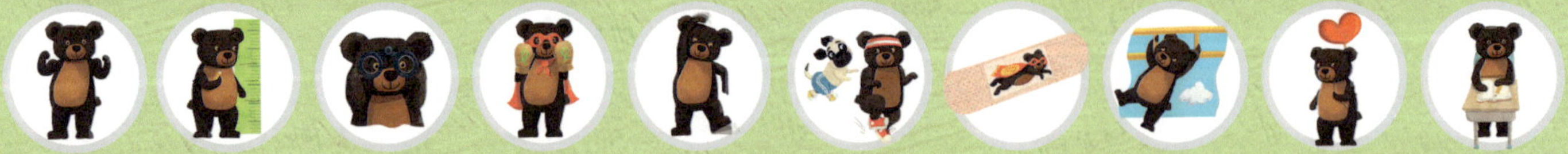

Hey, Boots the Bear,
what do you eat?

I eat yellow,
white, or even purple
CAULIFLOWER,
so I can grow healthy
and strong.

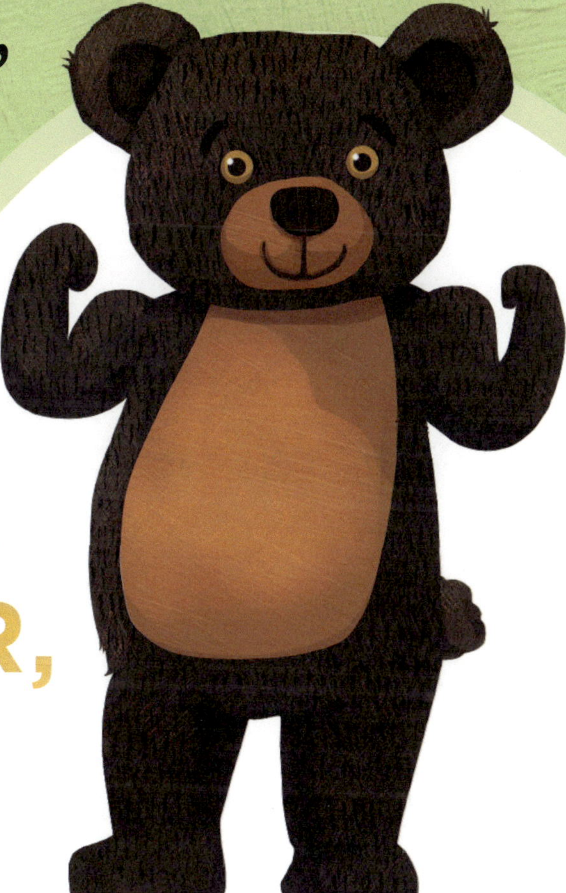

I eat

CORN

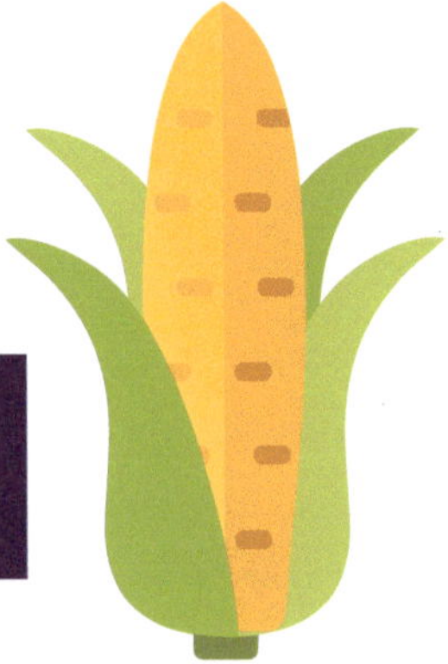

to help me leap,
twist, and dance.

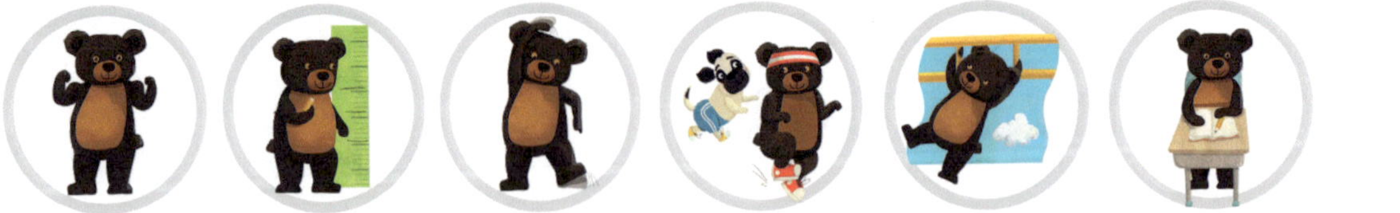

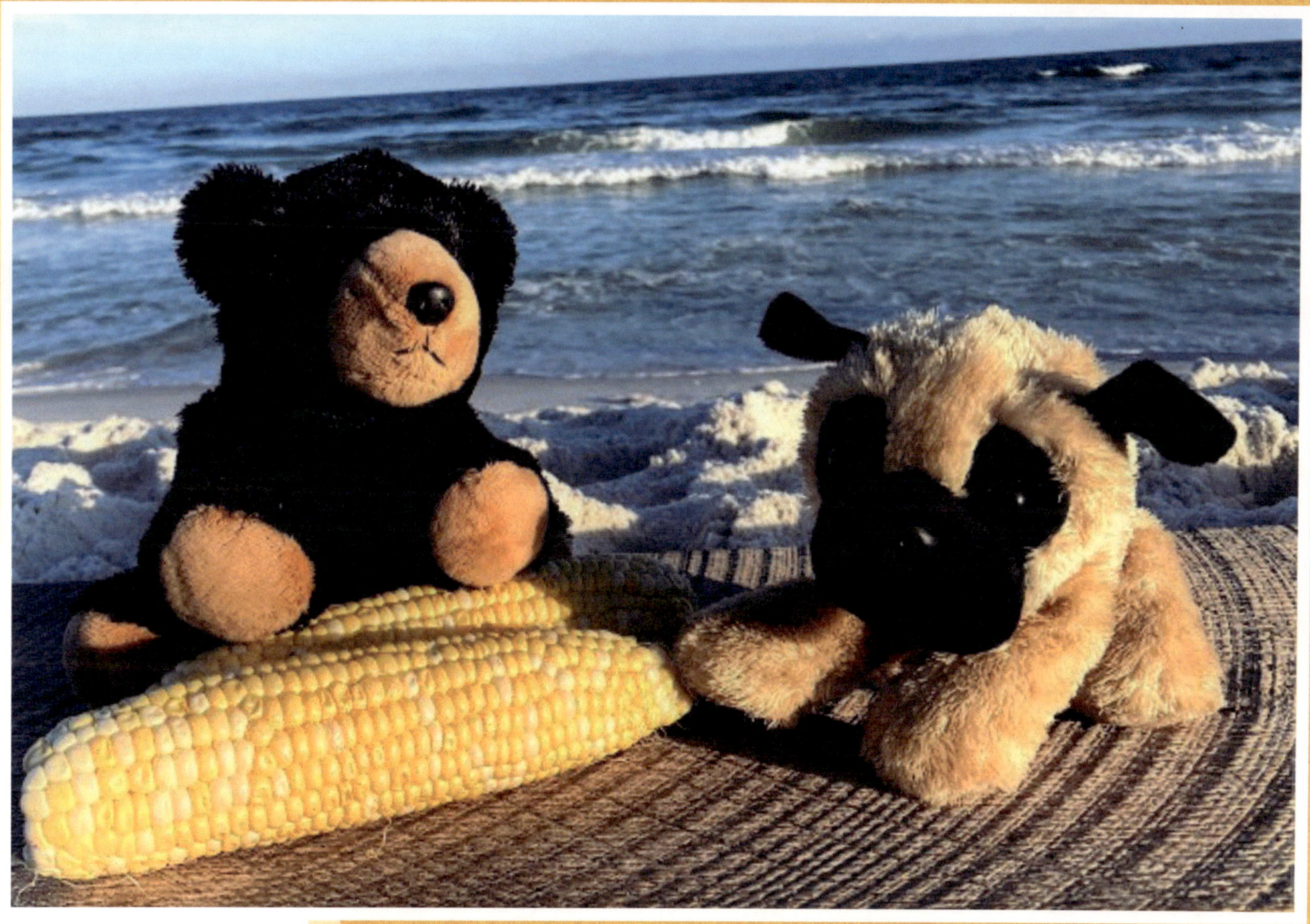

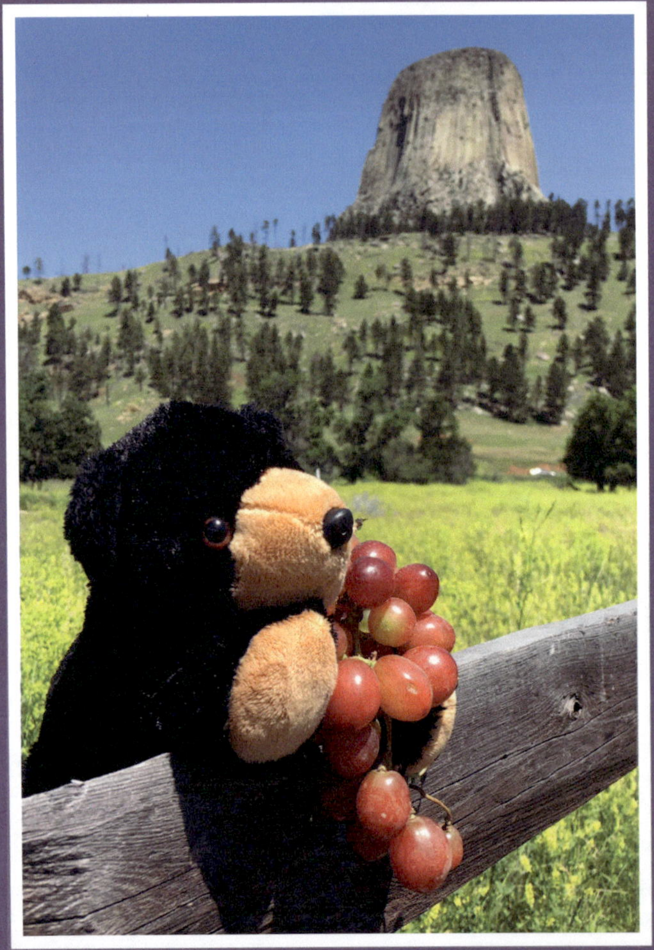

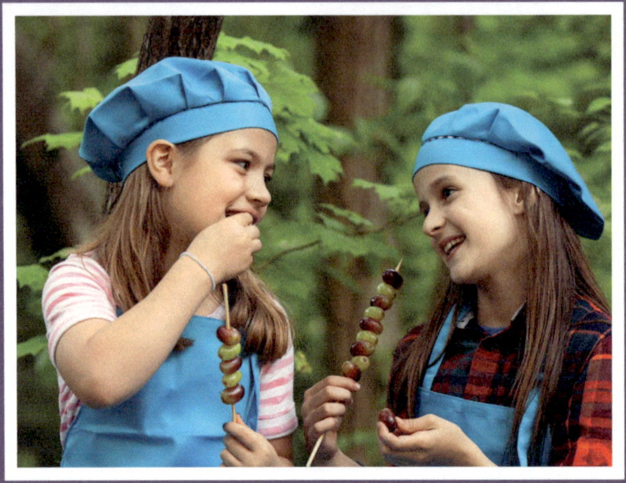

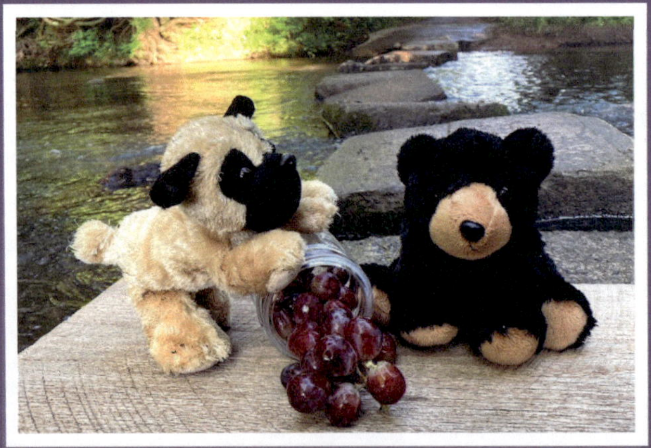

I eat

GRAPES

to help me run with lightning speed.

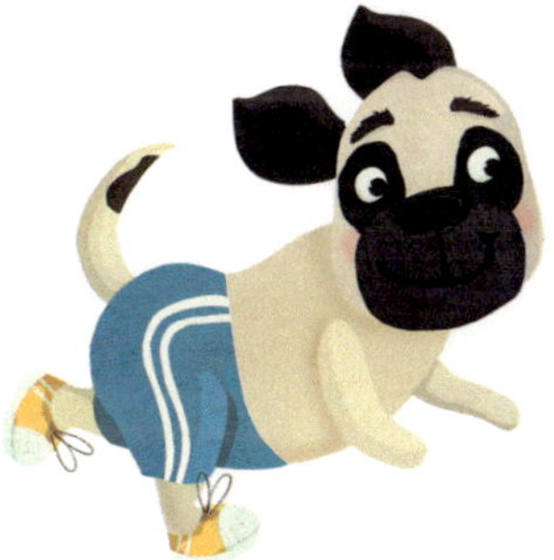

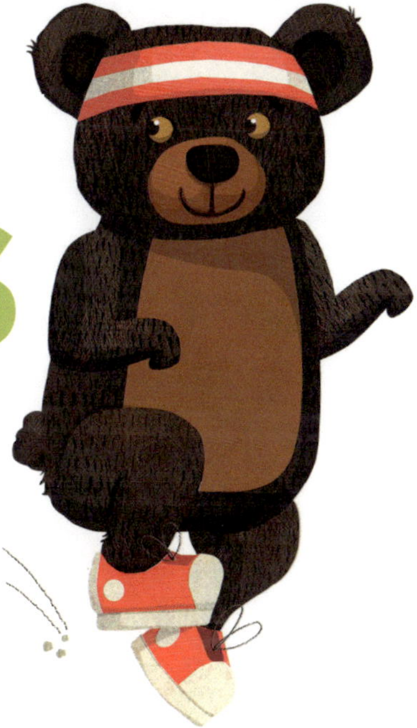

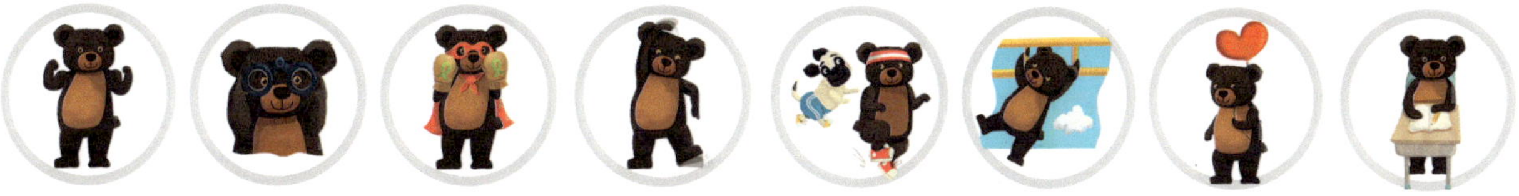

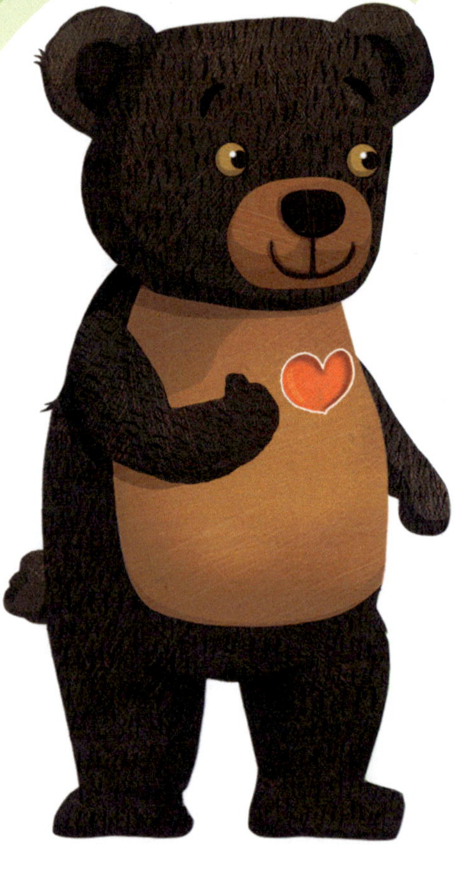

And I eat

GREEN BEANS

to help my heart beat strong.

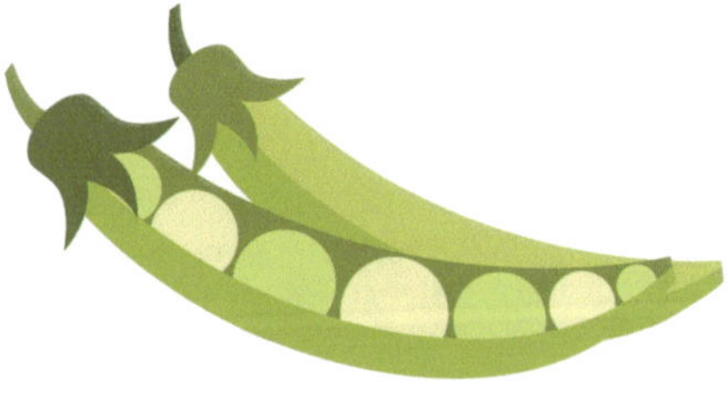

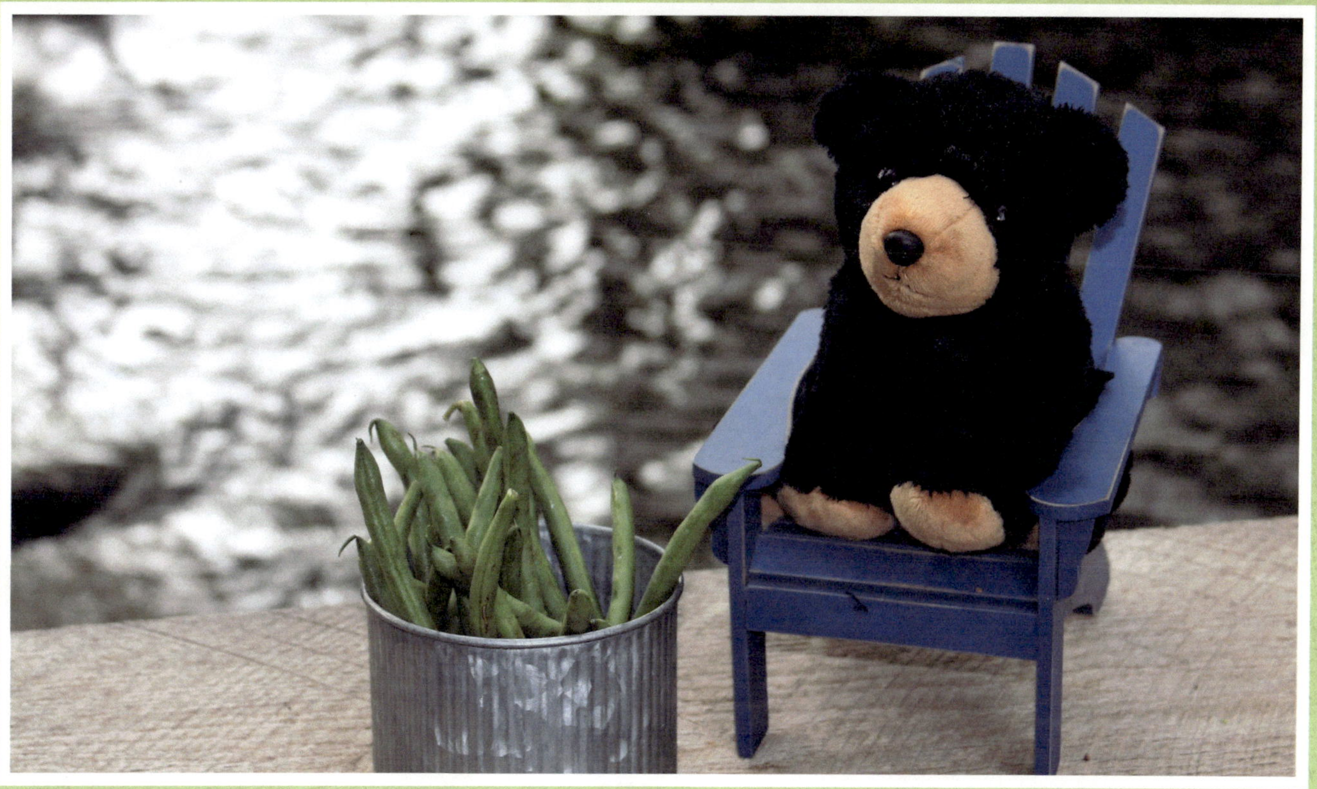

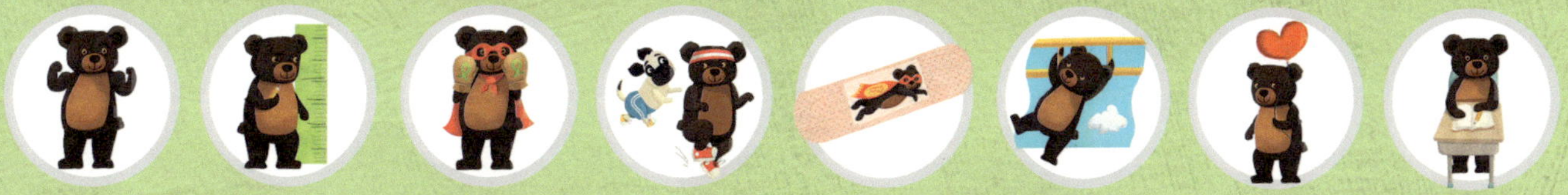

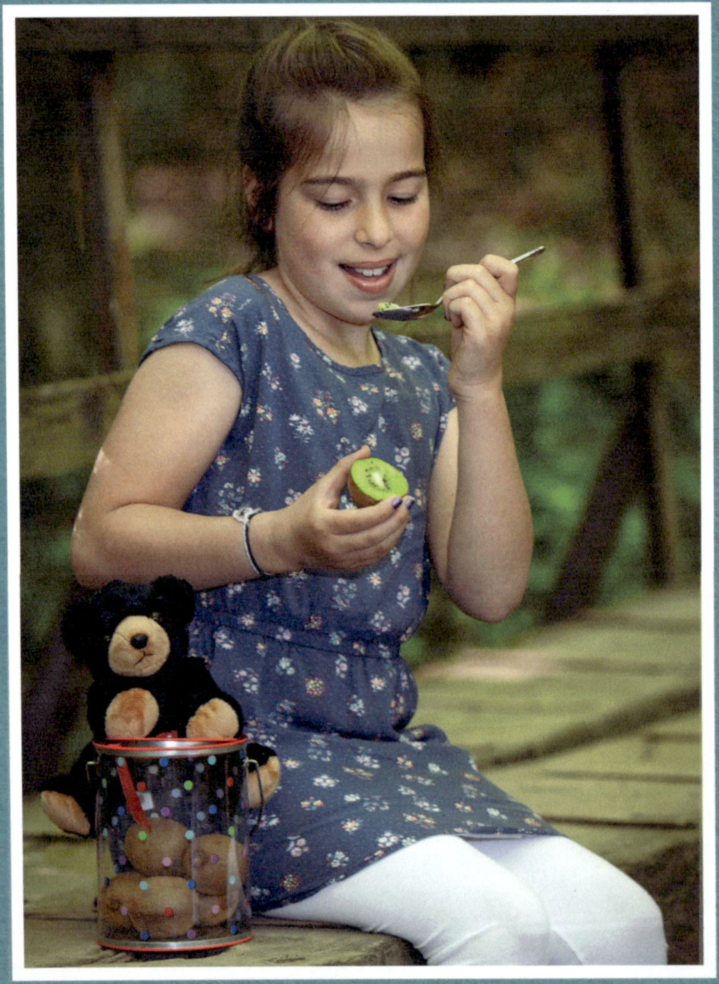

Hey, Boots the Bear, what do your friends eat?

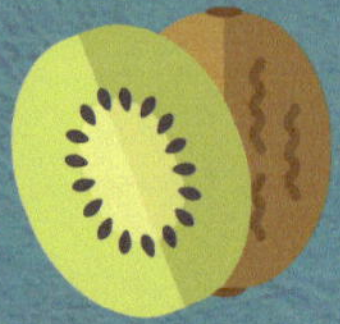

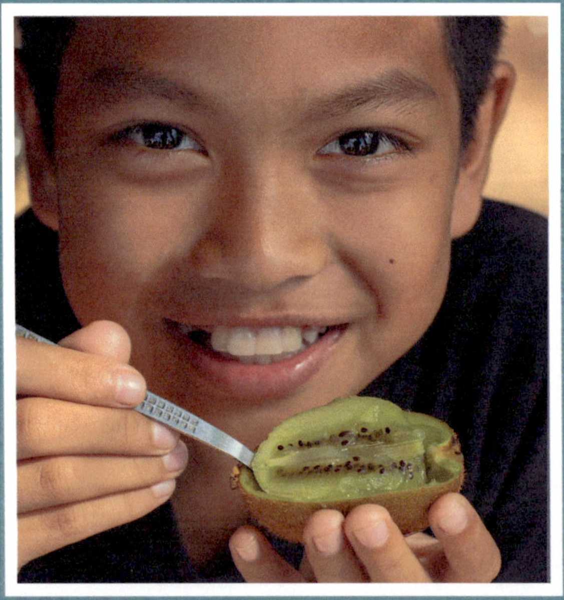

Beau the Bunny eats

KIWI

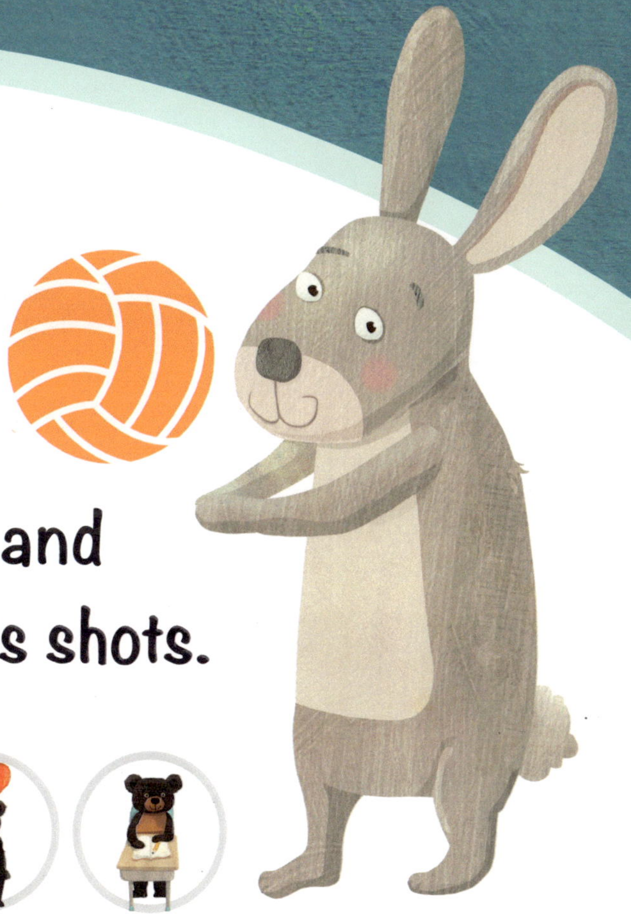

to help put more swoosh and sizzle in his super sports shots.

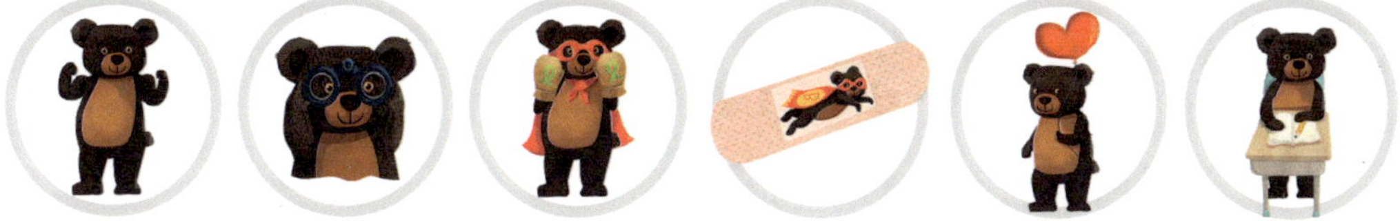

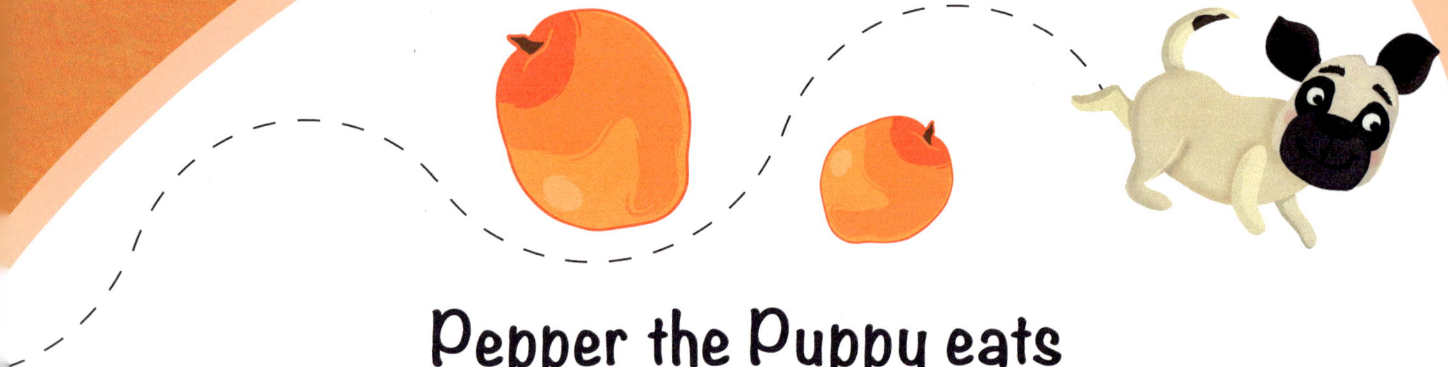

Pepper the Puppy eats

MANGOES

to help him make gigantic
leaps and jumps.

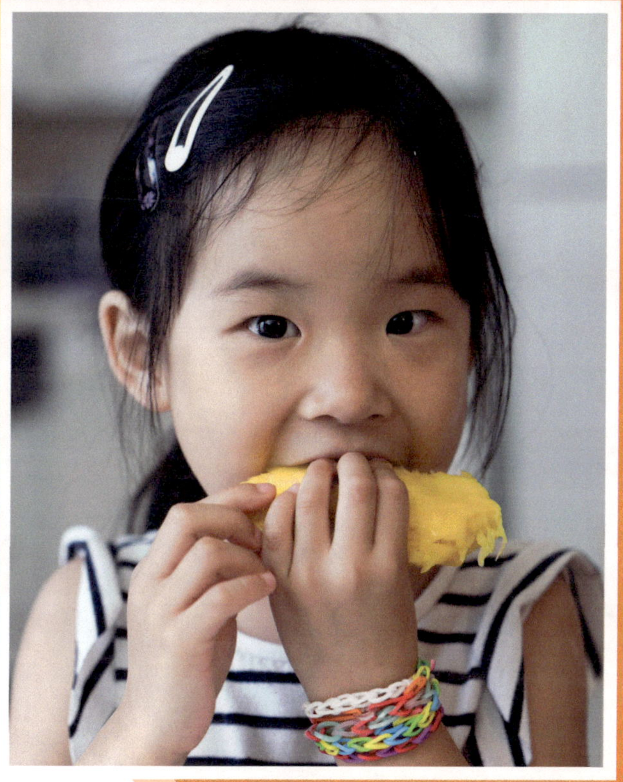

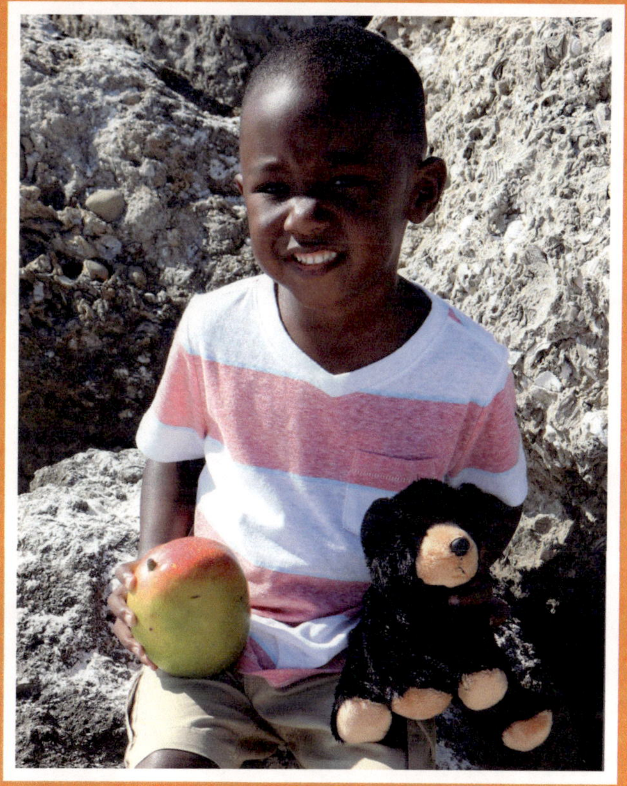

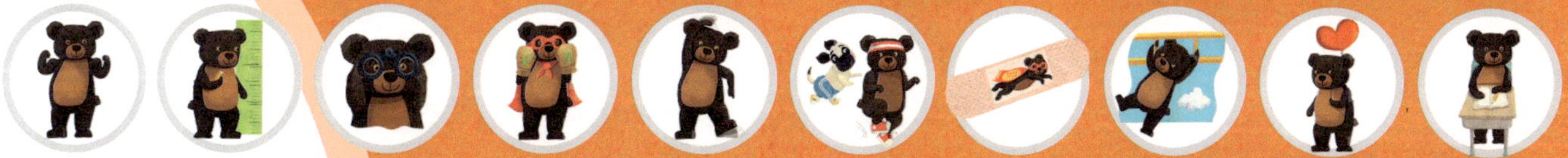

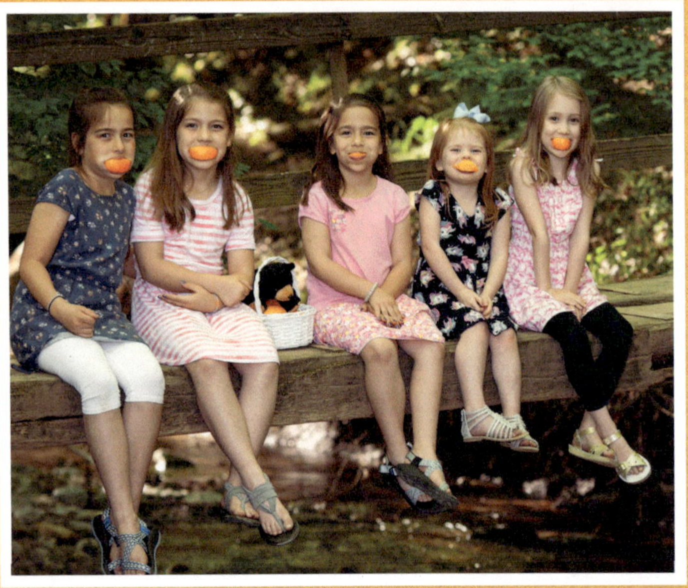
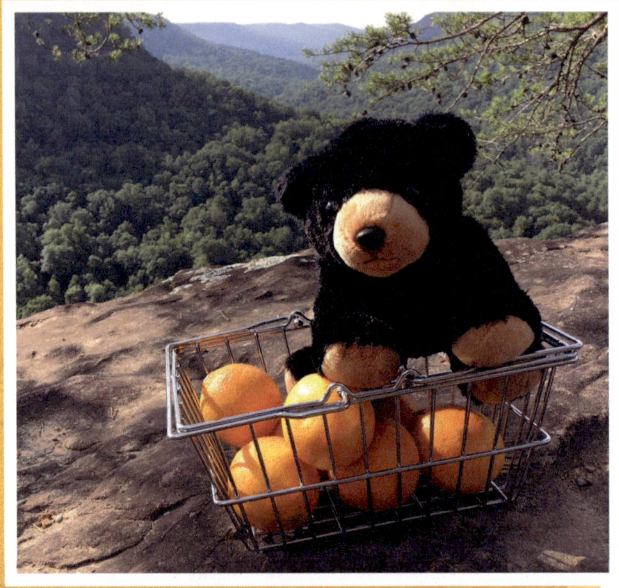
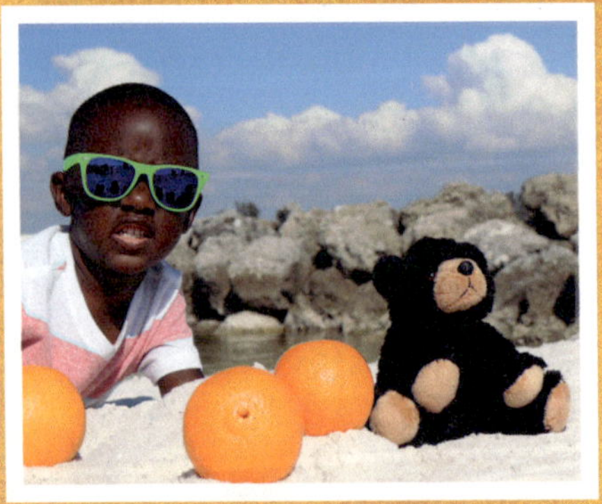
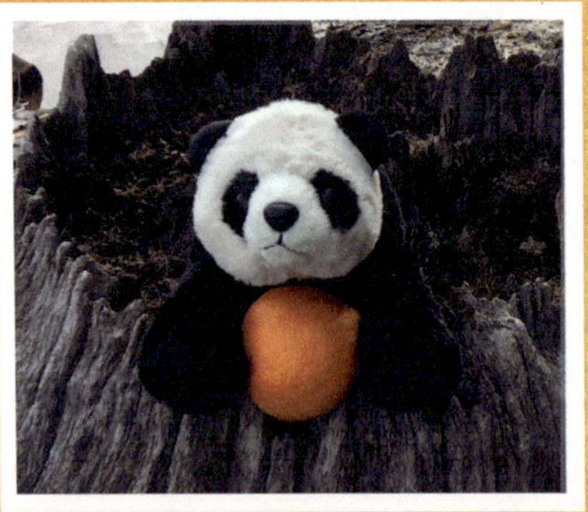
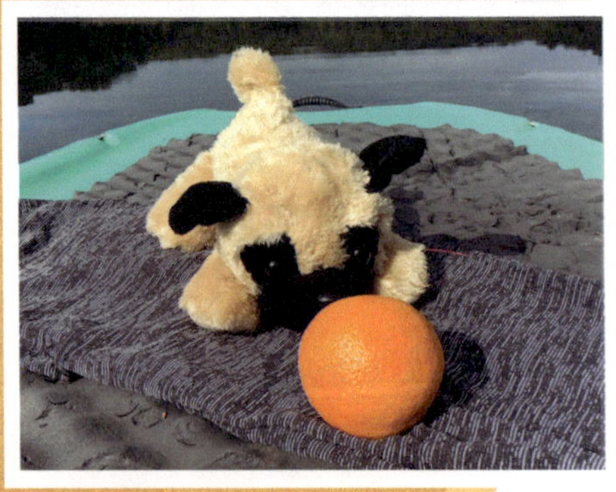

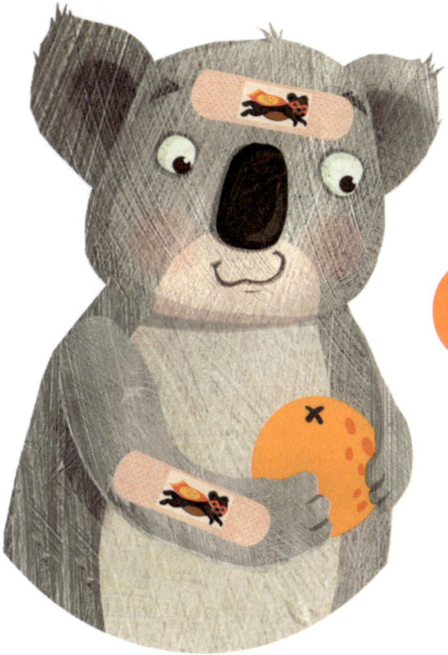

Kiwi the Koala eats

ORANGES

to feel better and
help heal his boo-boos.

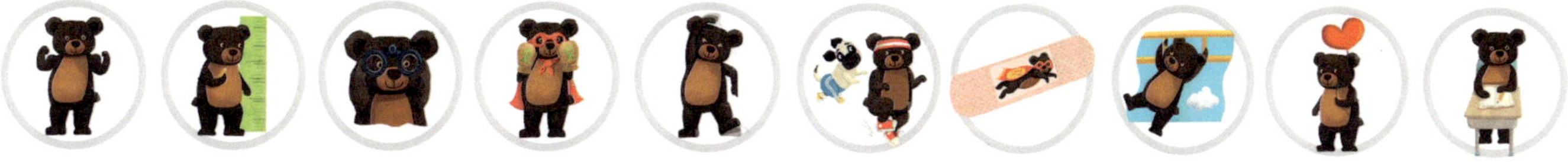

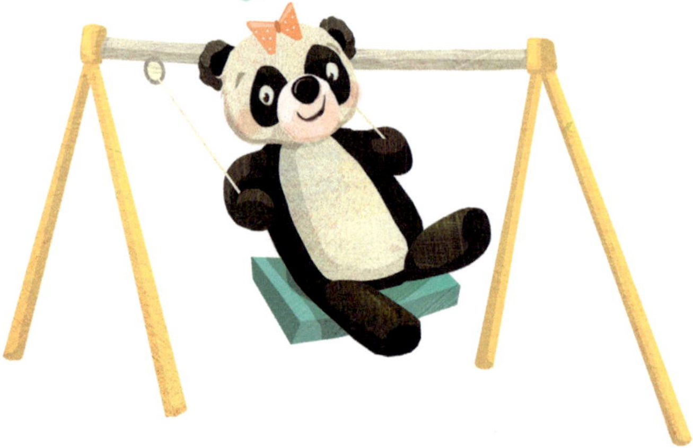

Pear the Panda eats

PEACHES

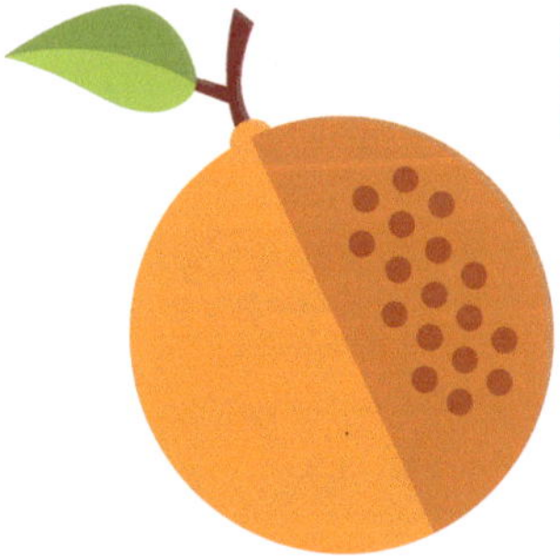

to help her swing and zing around the playground.

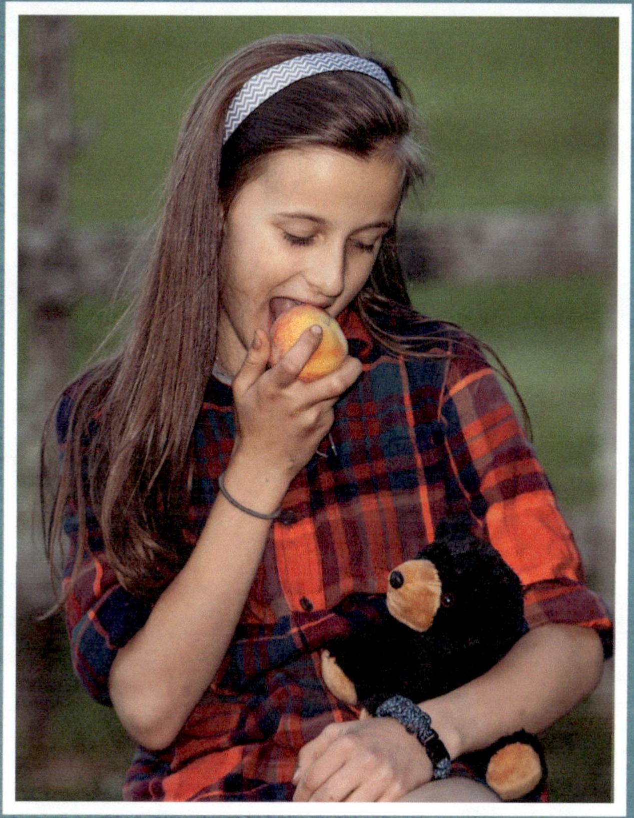

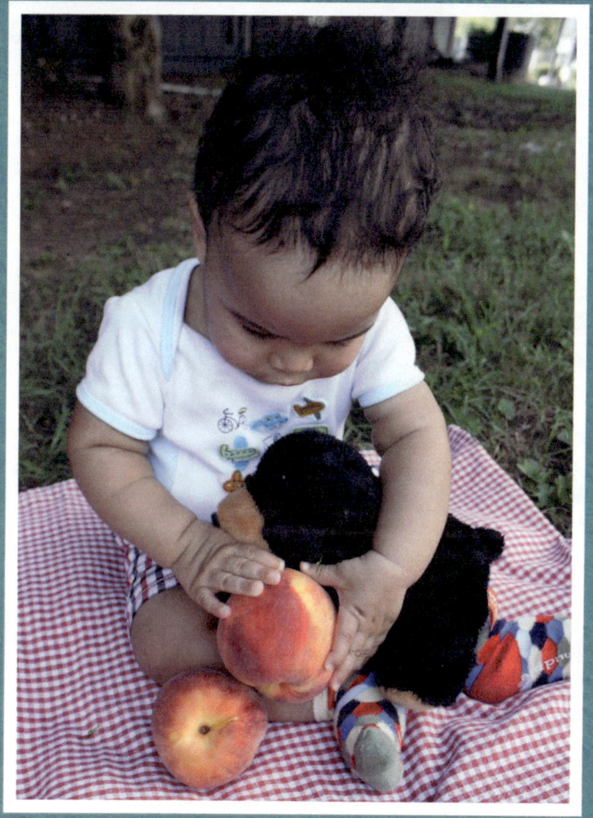

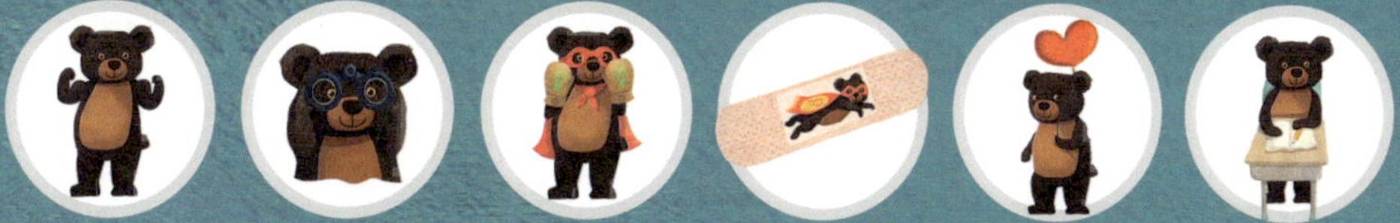

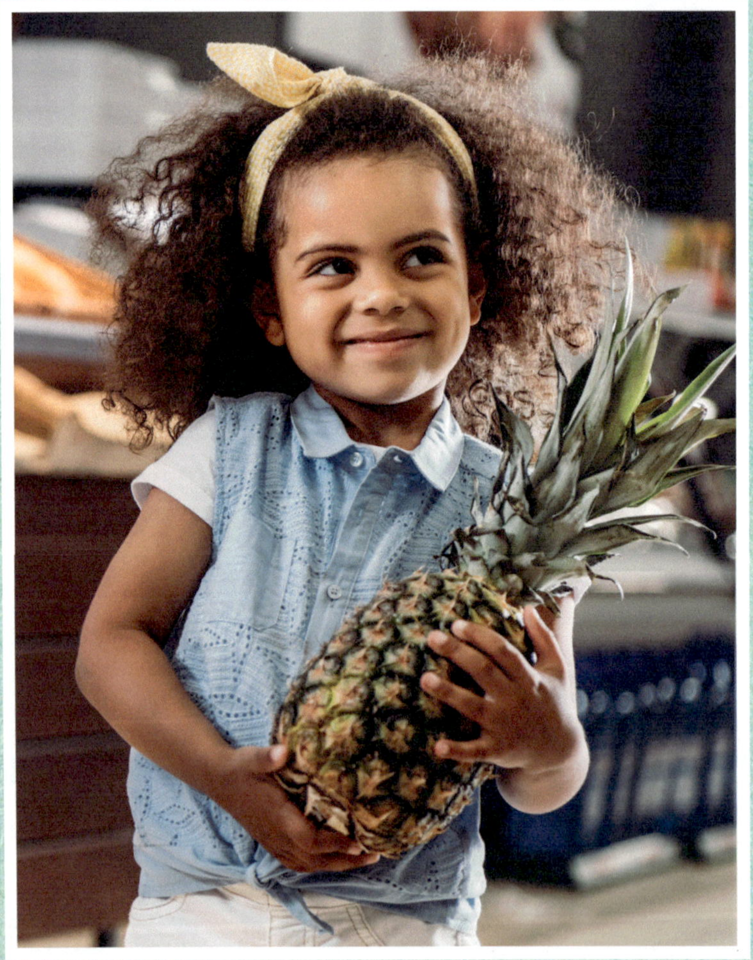
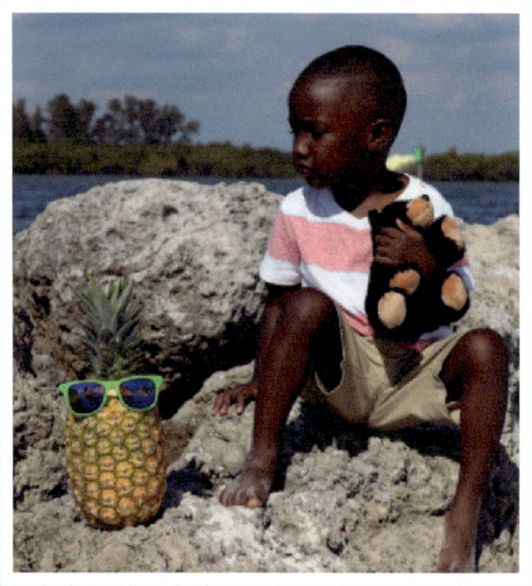
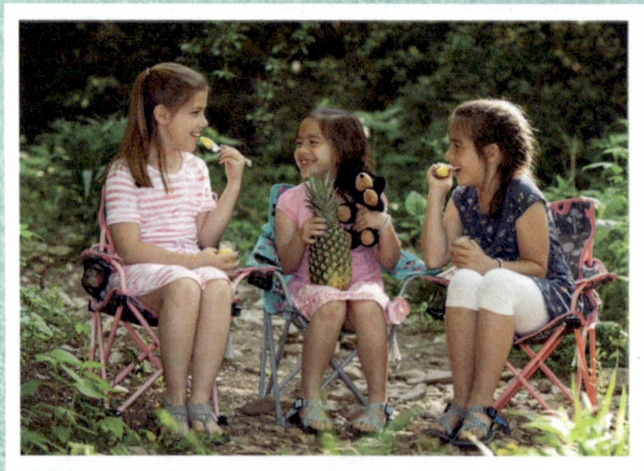

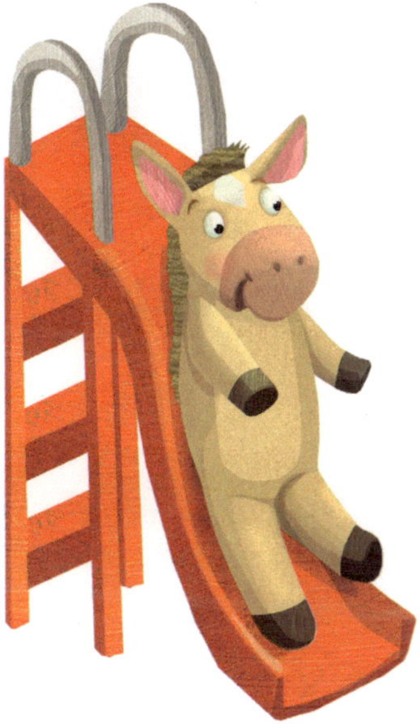

And Boots the Bear
and Huckleberry Horse eat

PINEAPPLE

to help them climb, crawl, and
slide through the playground.

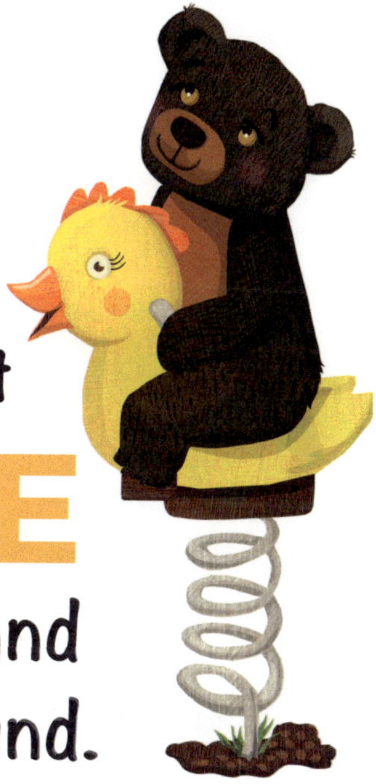

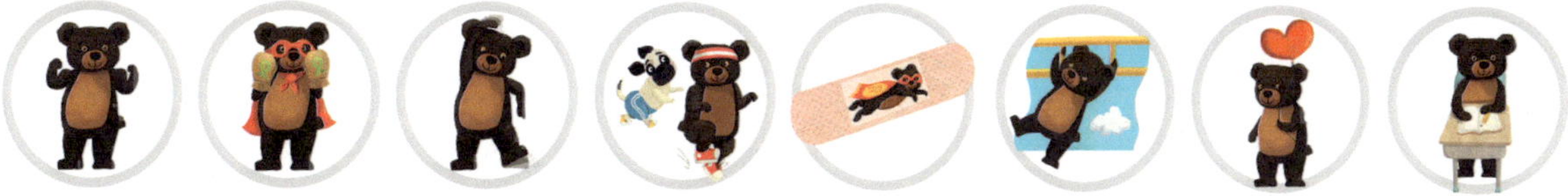

Hey, Boots the Bear,
what do you eat?

I eat

PLUMS

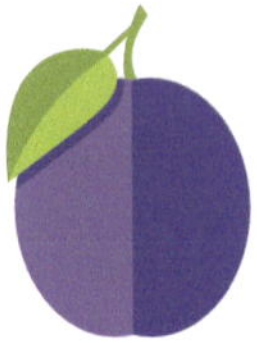

to help me match and
master my memory games.

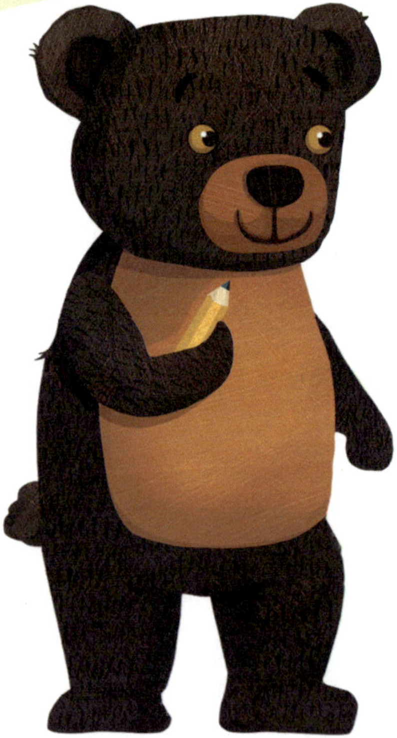

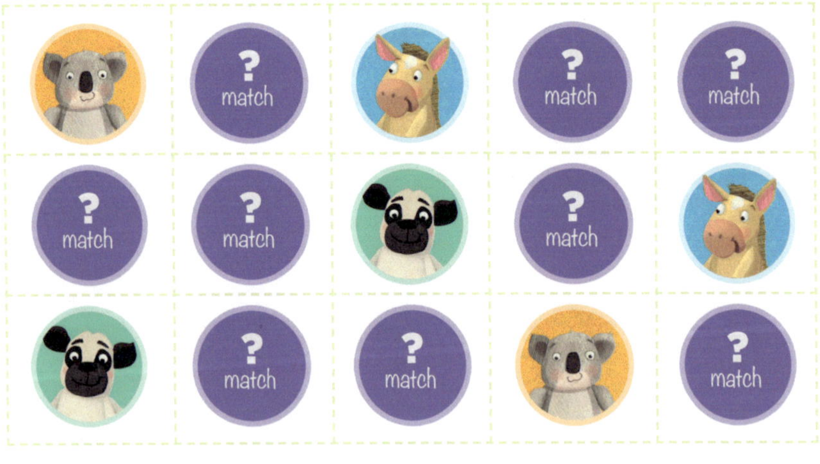

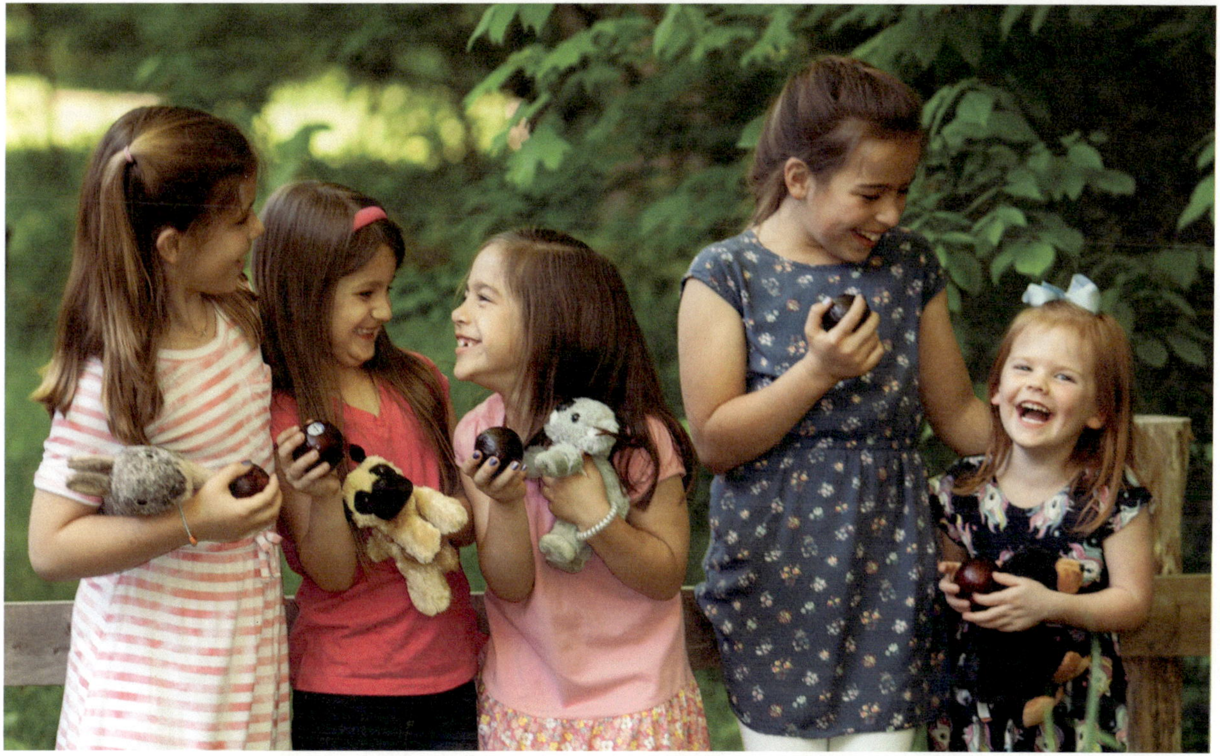

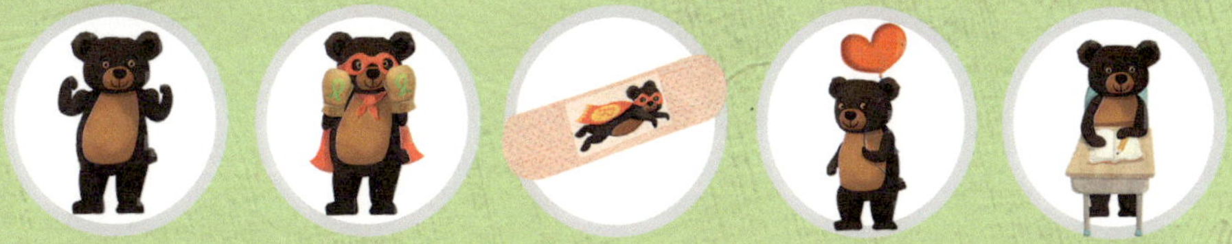

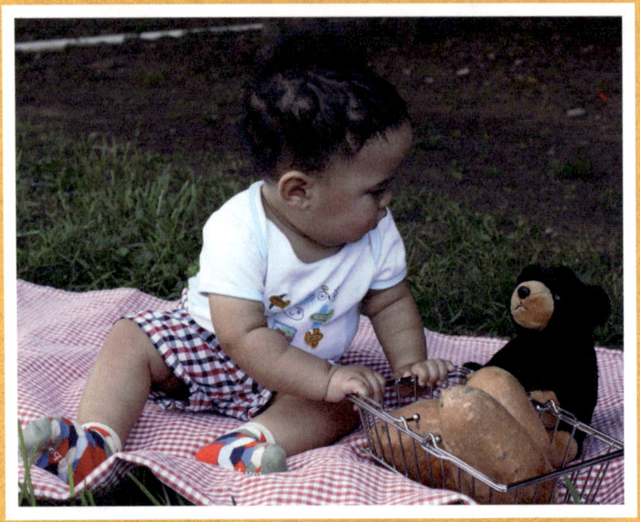
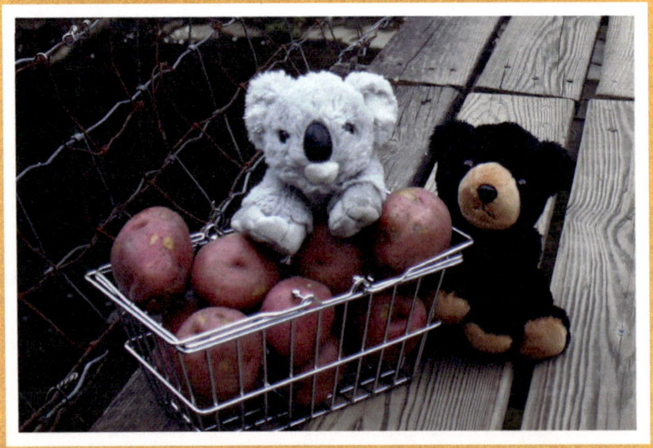
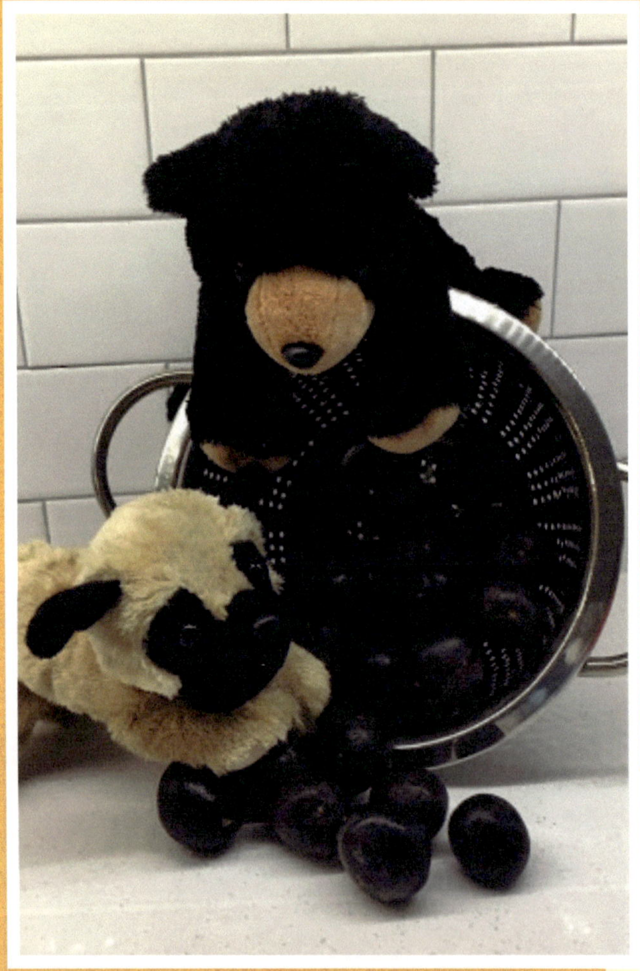

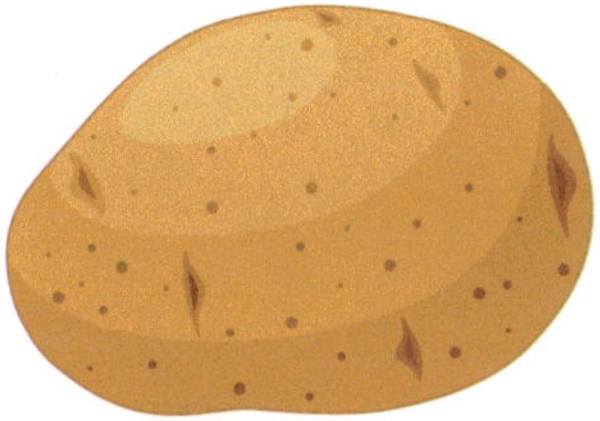

I eat all kinds of

POTATOES

WHITE, RED, PURPLE, AND SWEET

to help me grow big and strong.

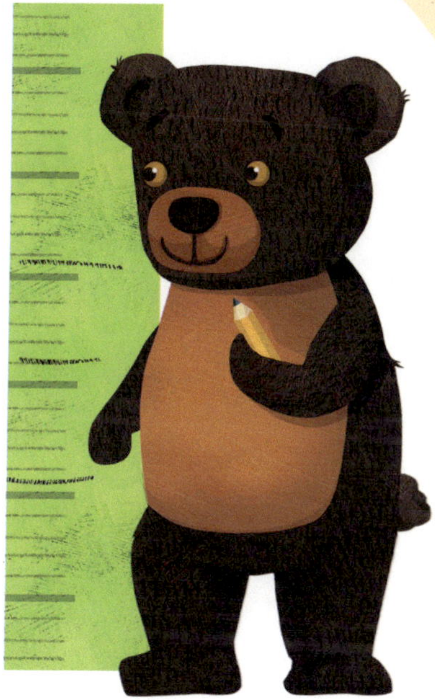

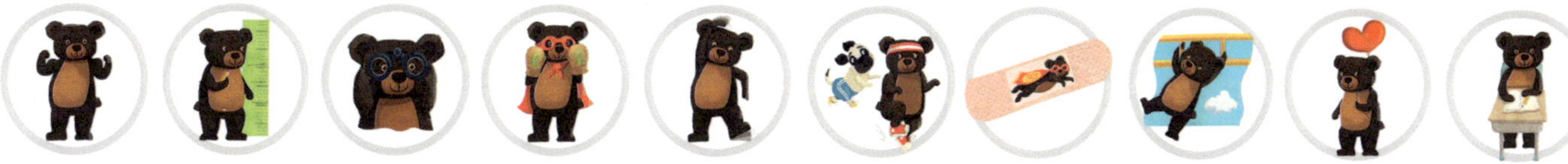

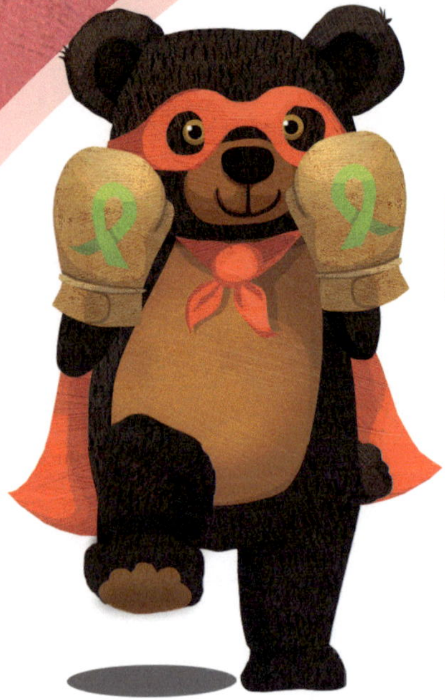

I eat 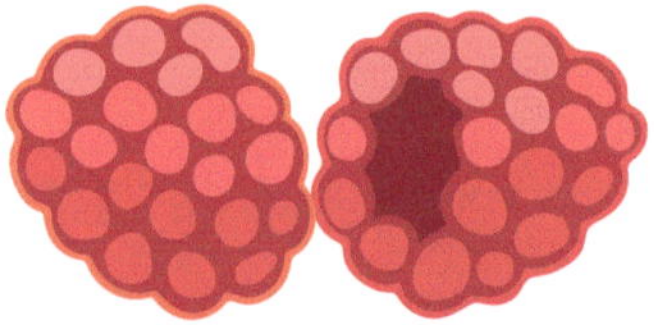

RASPBERRIES

to help make
mighty ninja kicks.

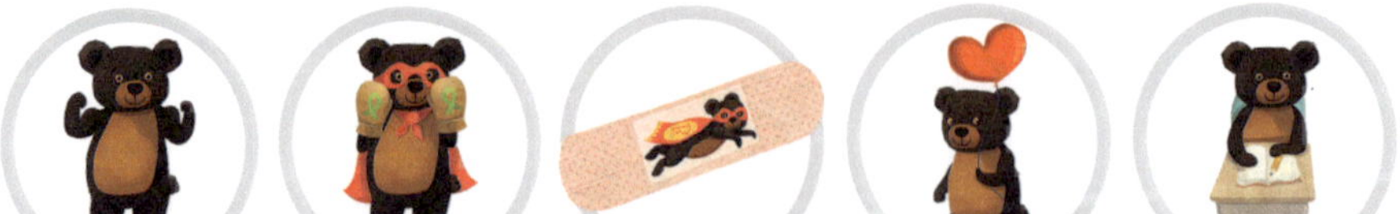

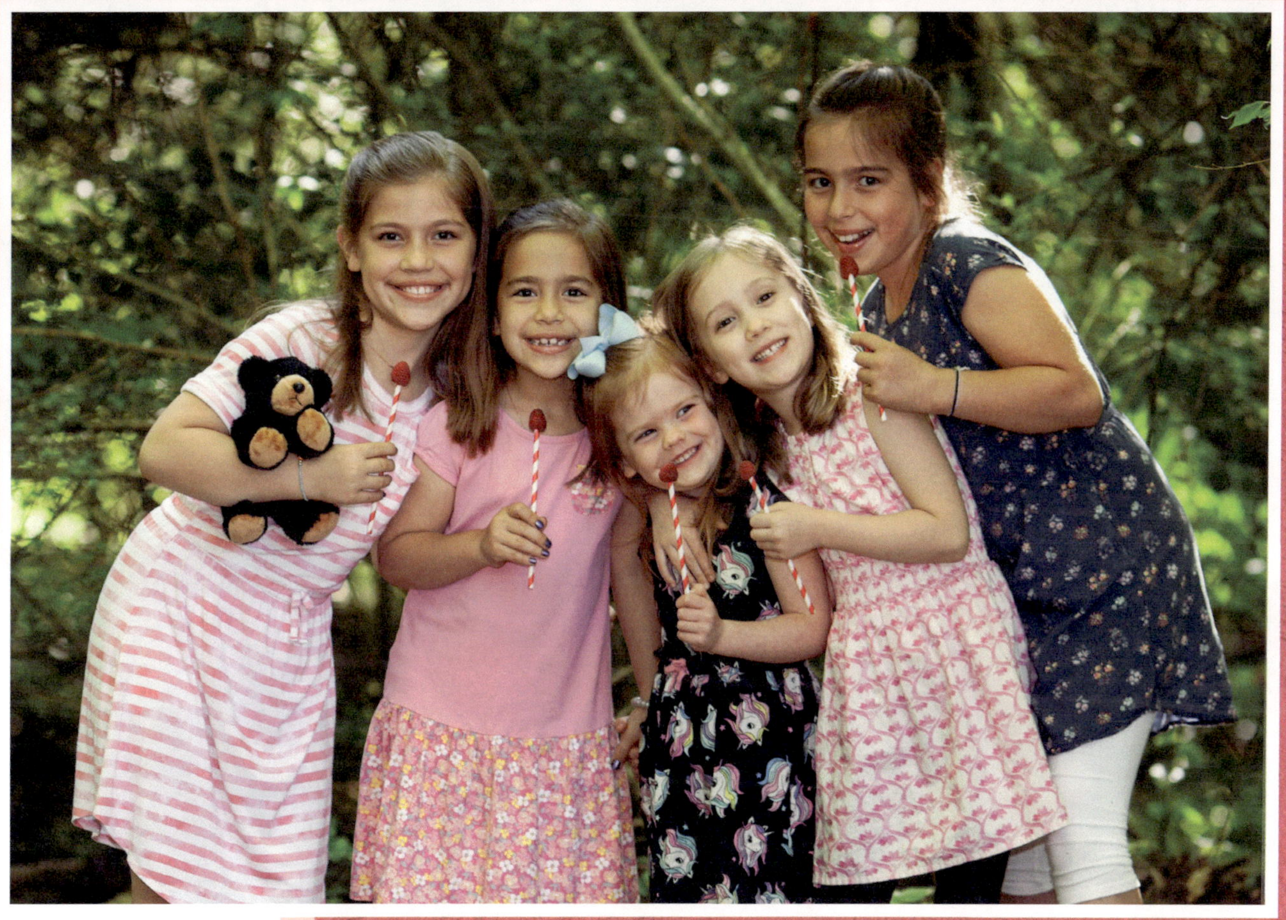

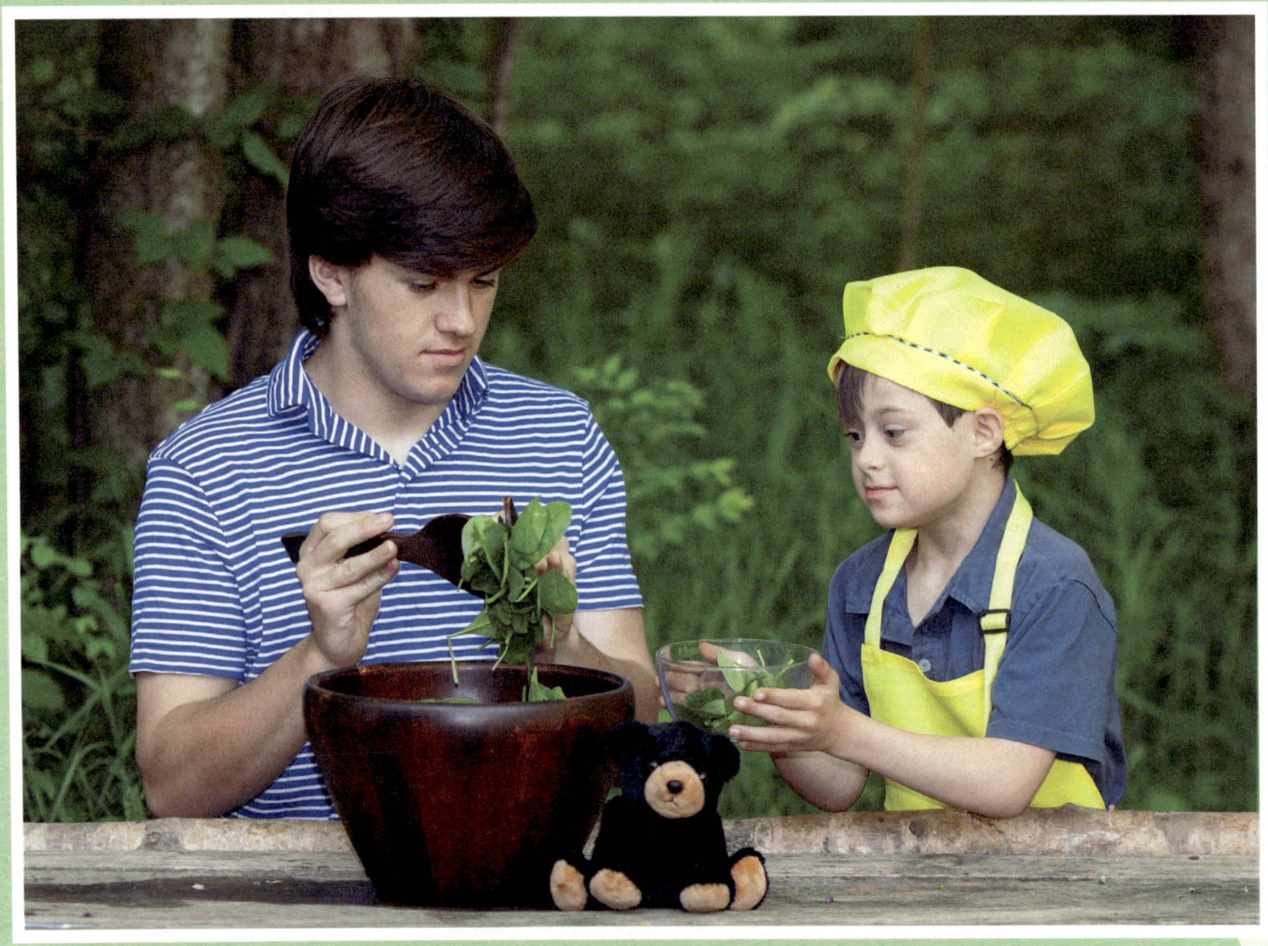

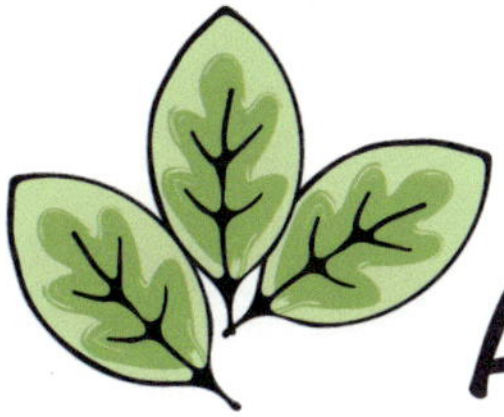

And I eat

SPINACH

to help me build strong muscles.

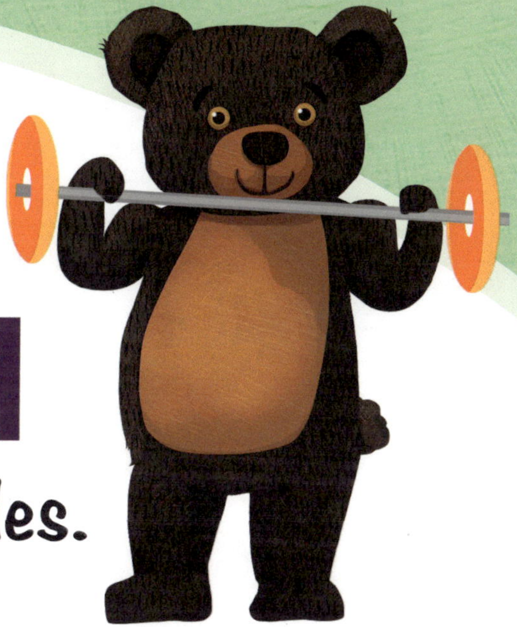

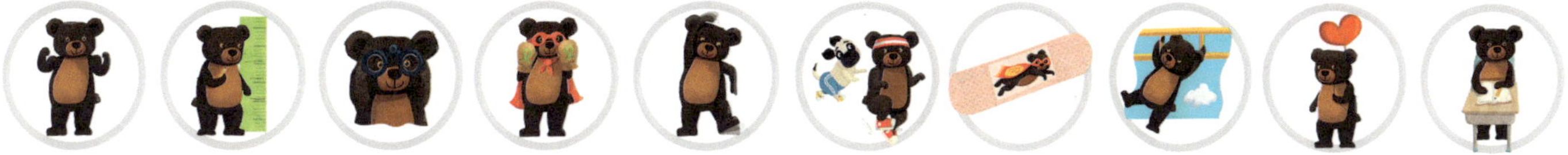

Hey, Boots the Bear,
what do your
friends eat?

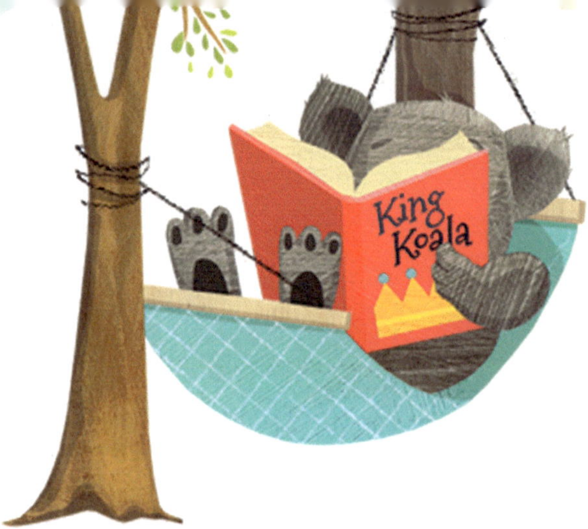

Kiwi the Koala eats

STRAWBERRIES

to help keep his brain bright and smart.

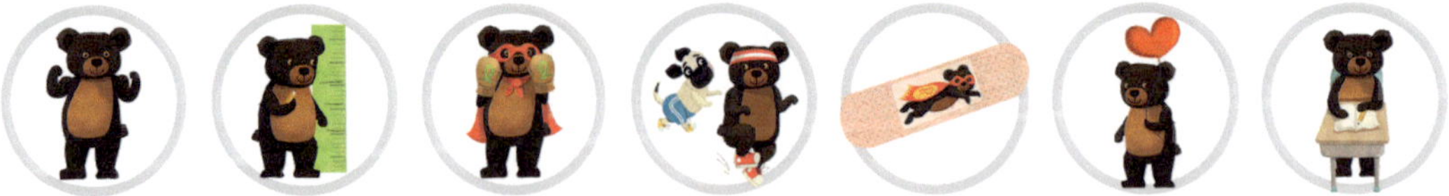

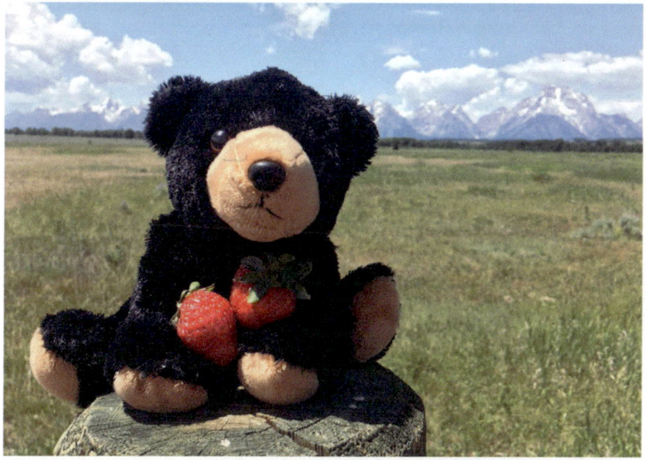

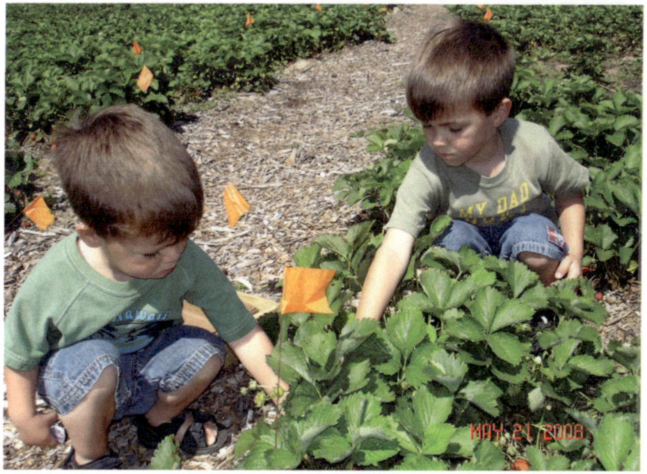
MY DAD
MAY 21 2008

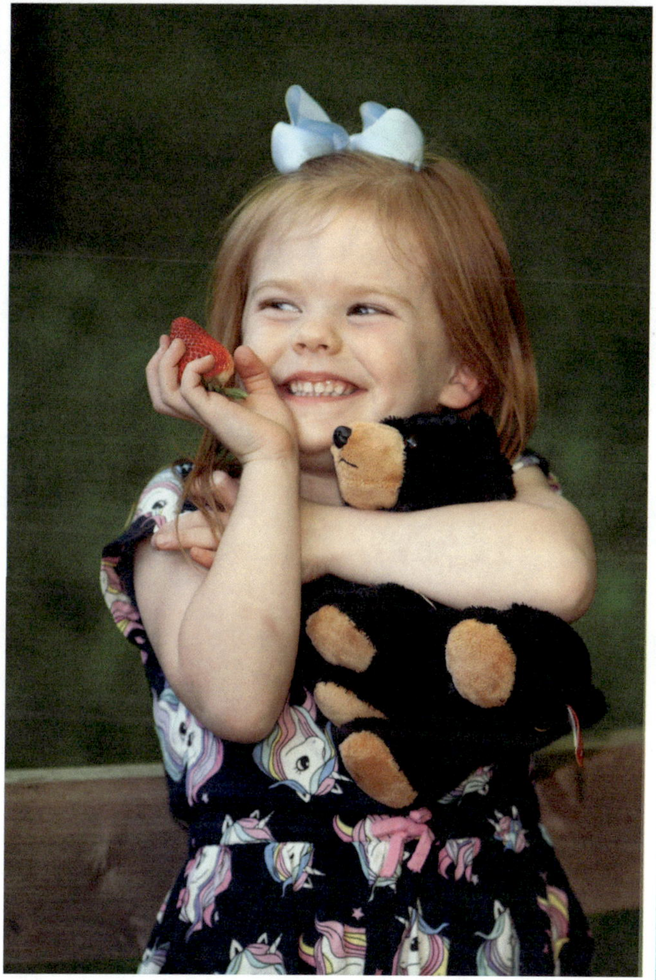

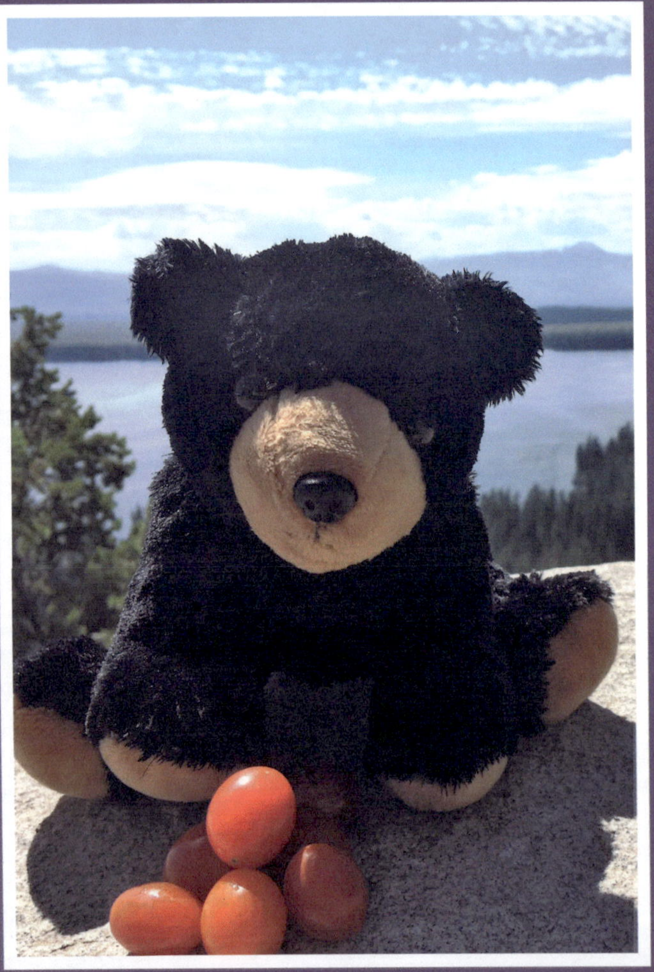
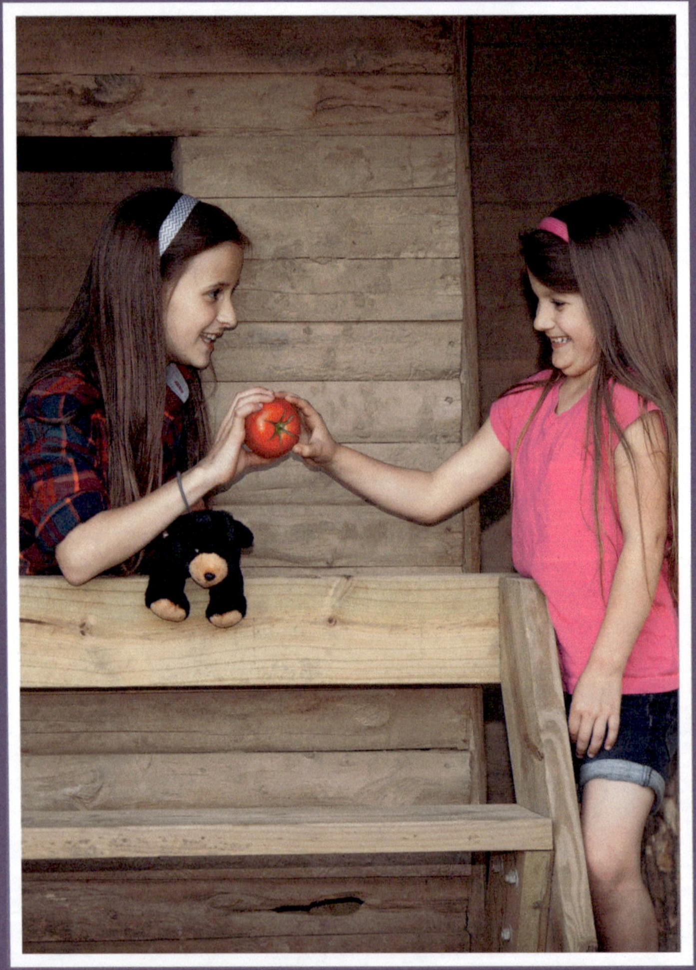

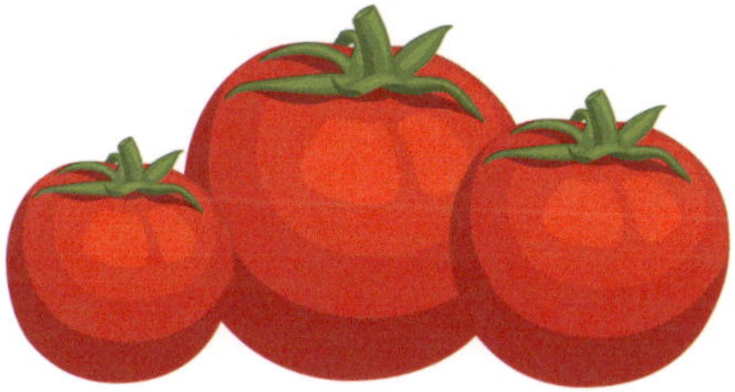

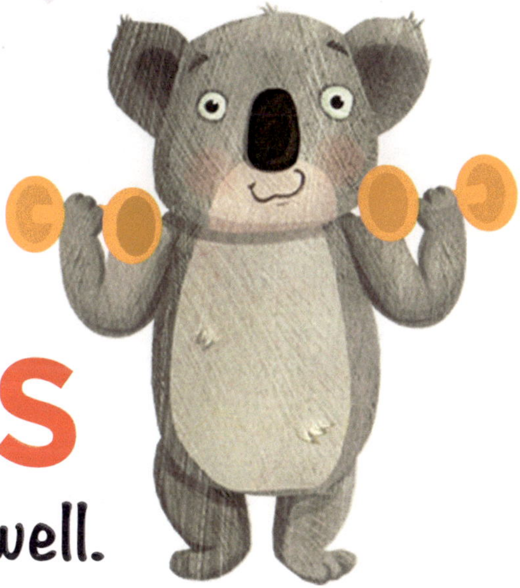

Kiwi the Koala also eats

TOMATOES

to help keep his body fit and well.

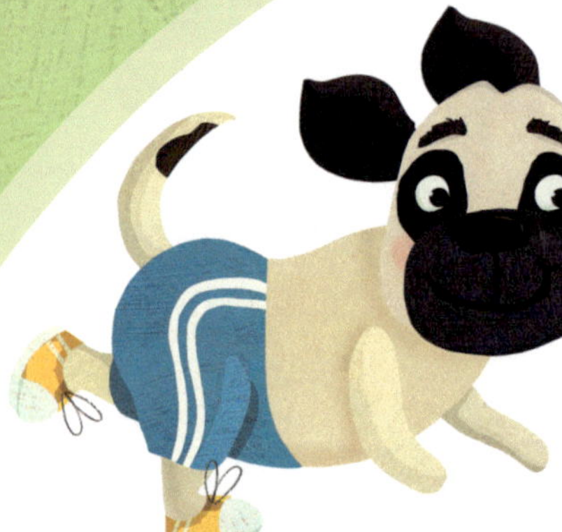

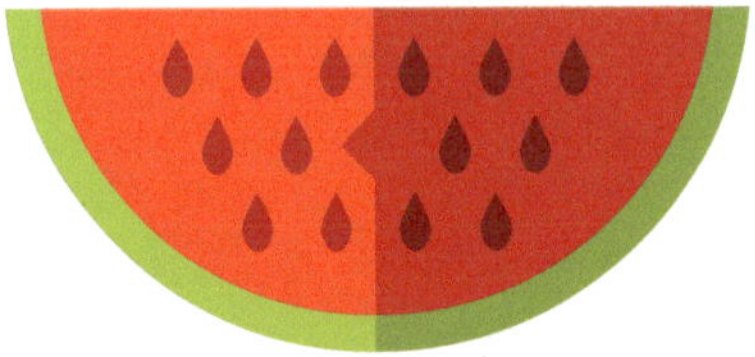

Pepper the Puppy eats

WATERMELON

to help him race around the
track with super speed.

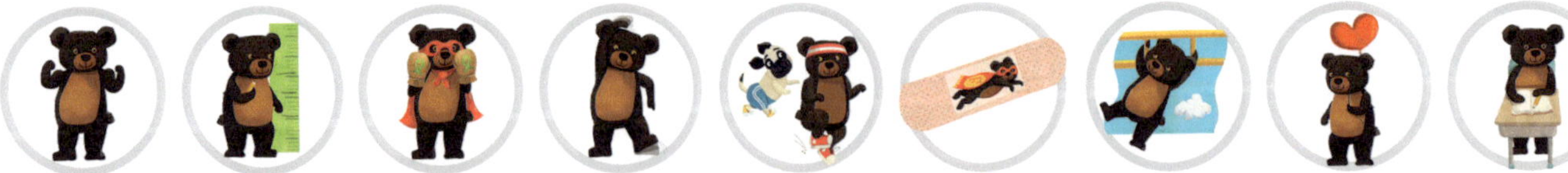

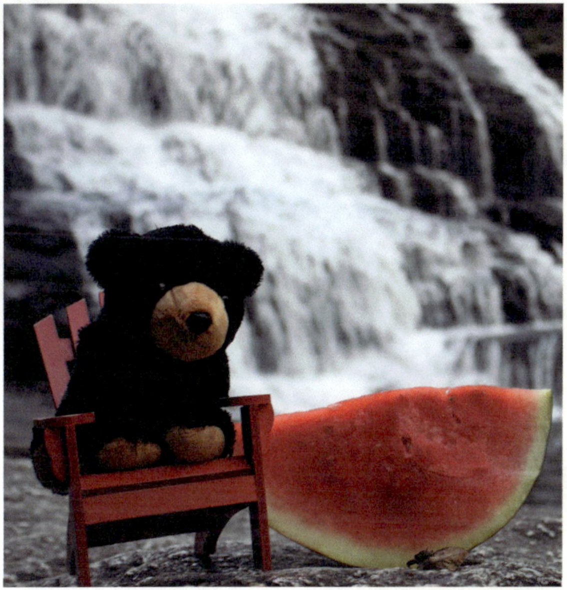
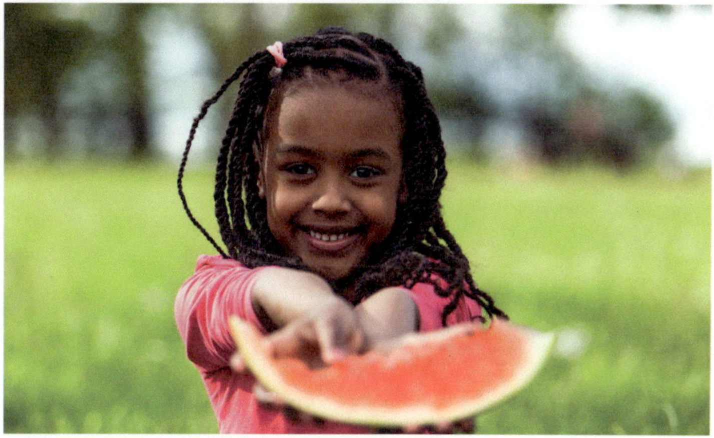
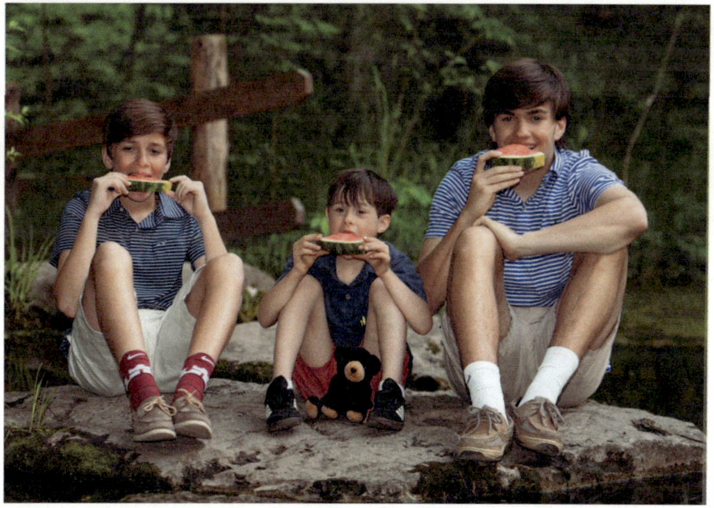

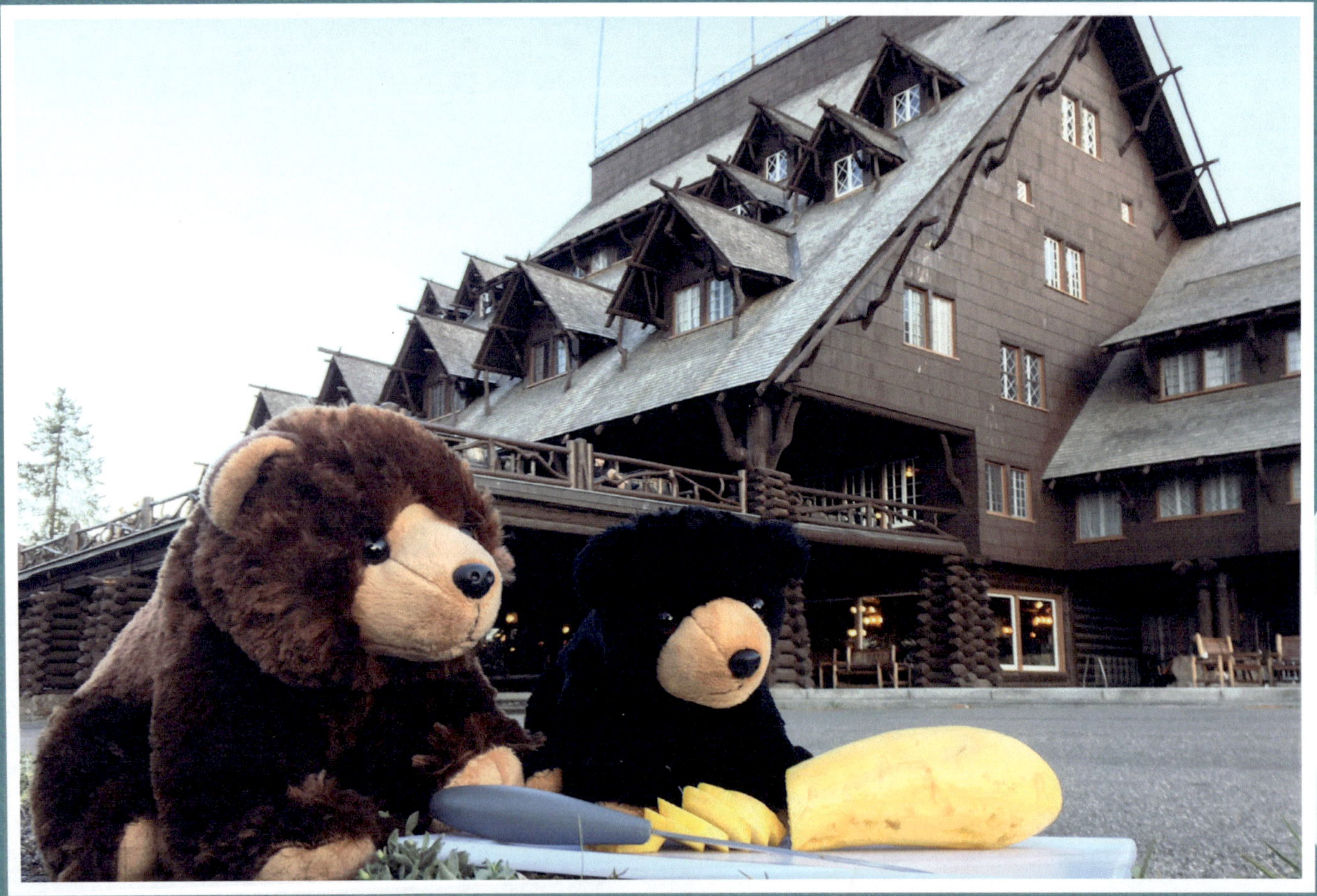

cha-cha-cah

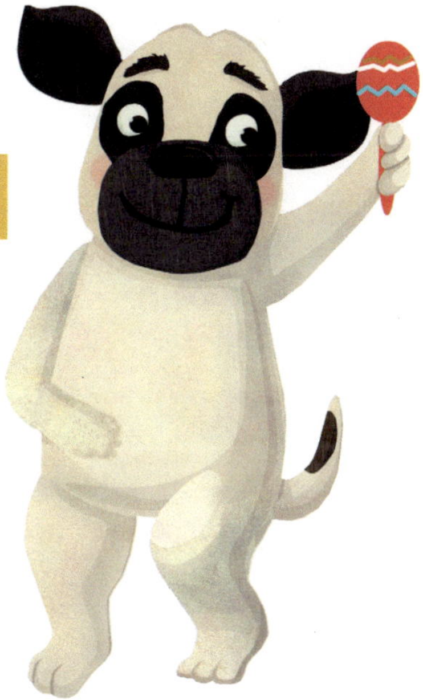

Pepper the Puppy eats

YELLOW SQUASH

to help his heart beat strong as
his feet dance, dance, dance.

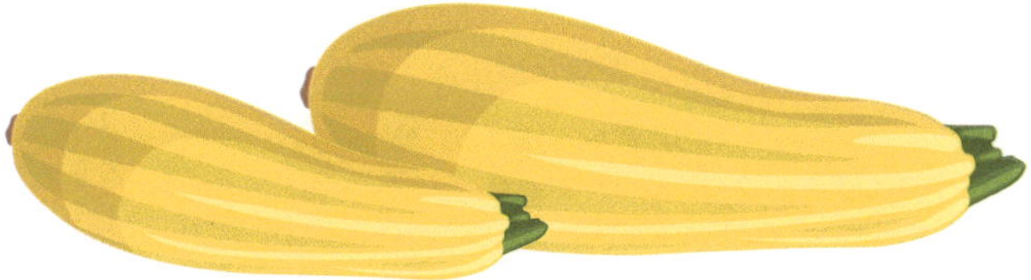

And finally, Boots the Bear,
what do you eat?

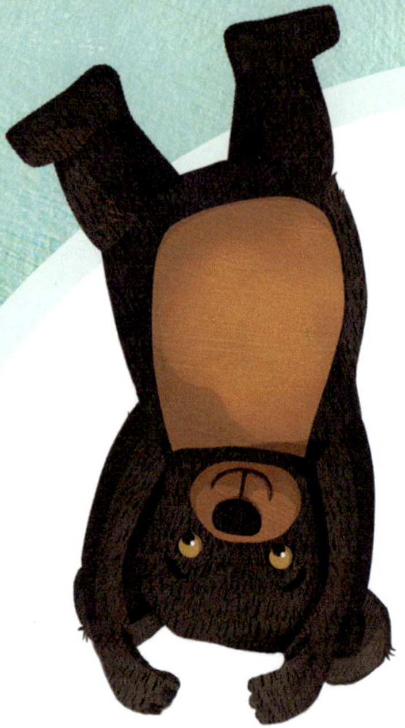

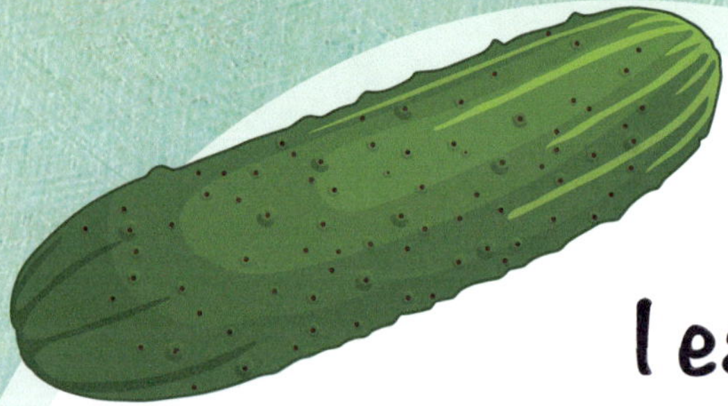

I eat

ZUCCHINI

to help me do somersaults,
jumping jacks, and headstands.

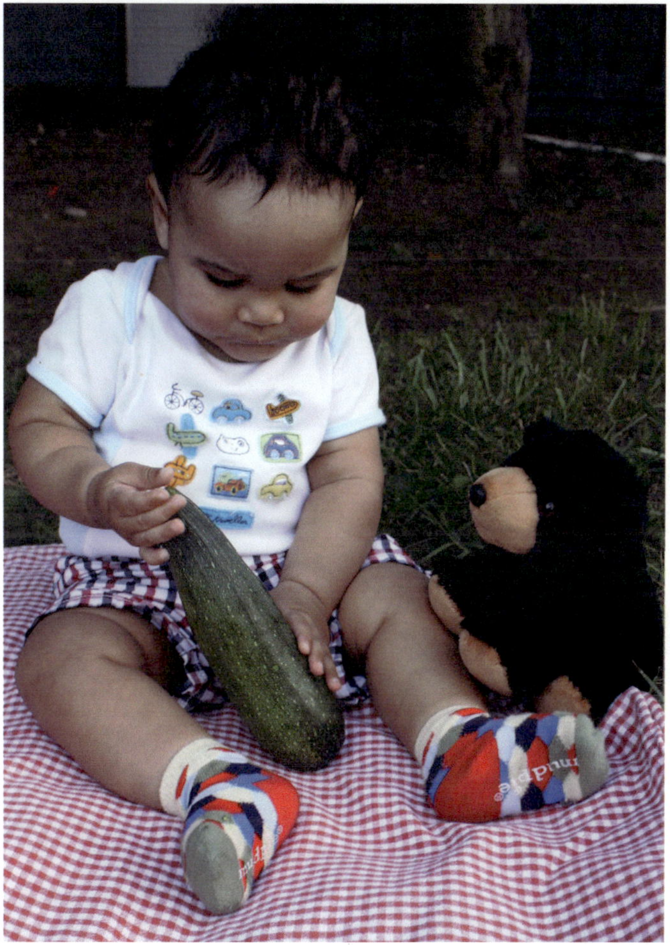

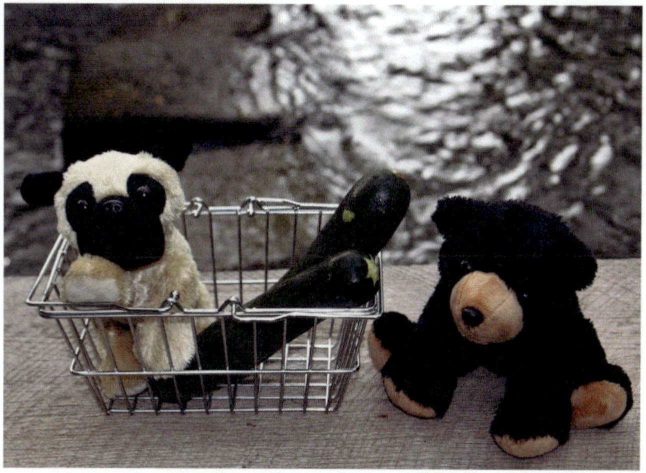

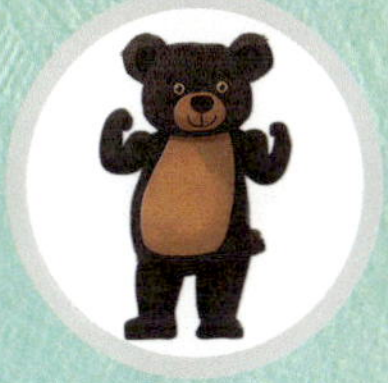

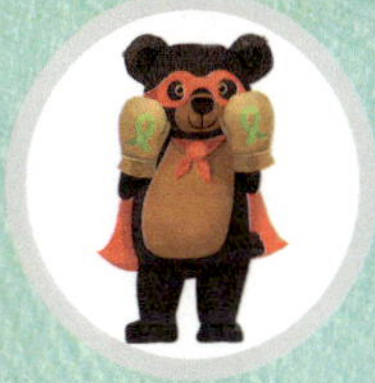

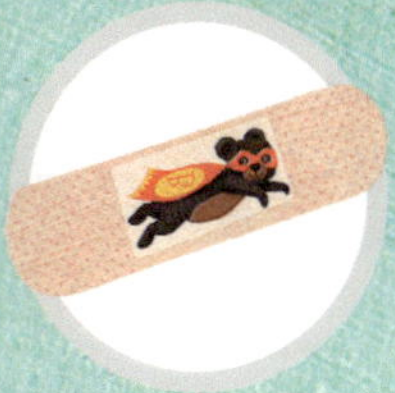

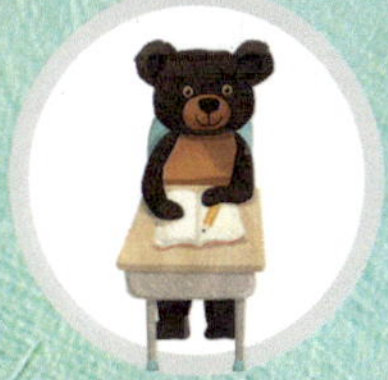

Boots and friends add color to their plates each day by eating from the FIVE Color Groups of Fruits and Vegetables.

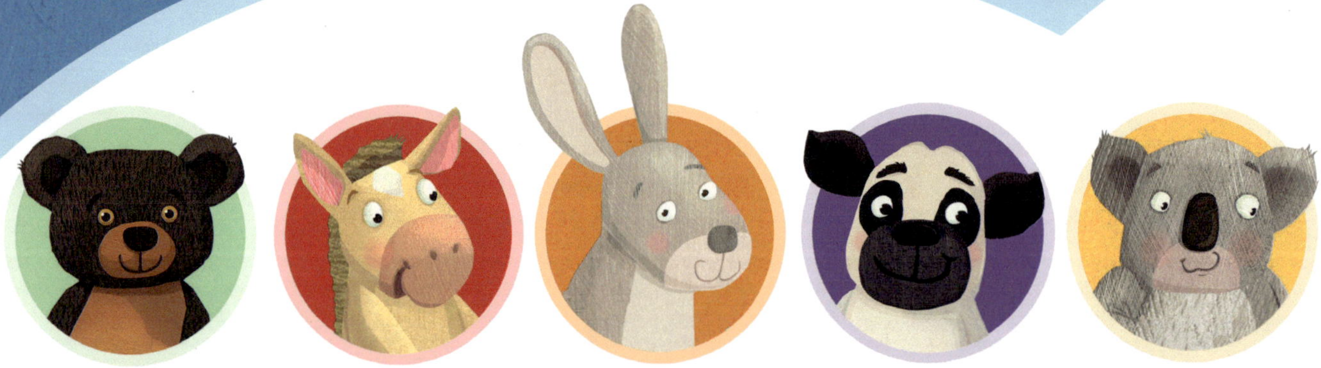

GREEN

RED

YELLOW/ ORANGE

BLUE/ PURPLE

WHITE

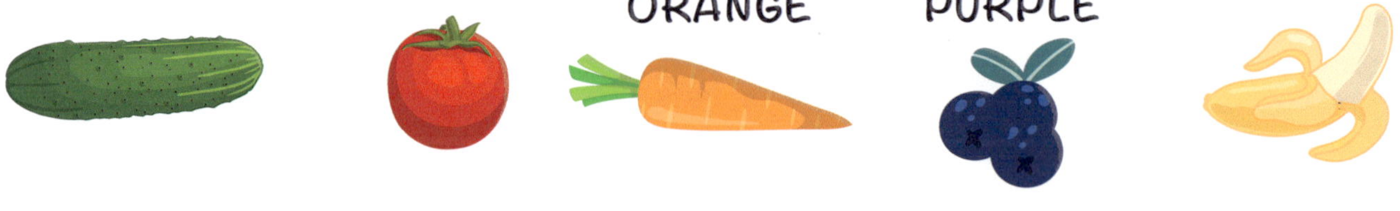

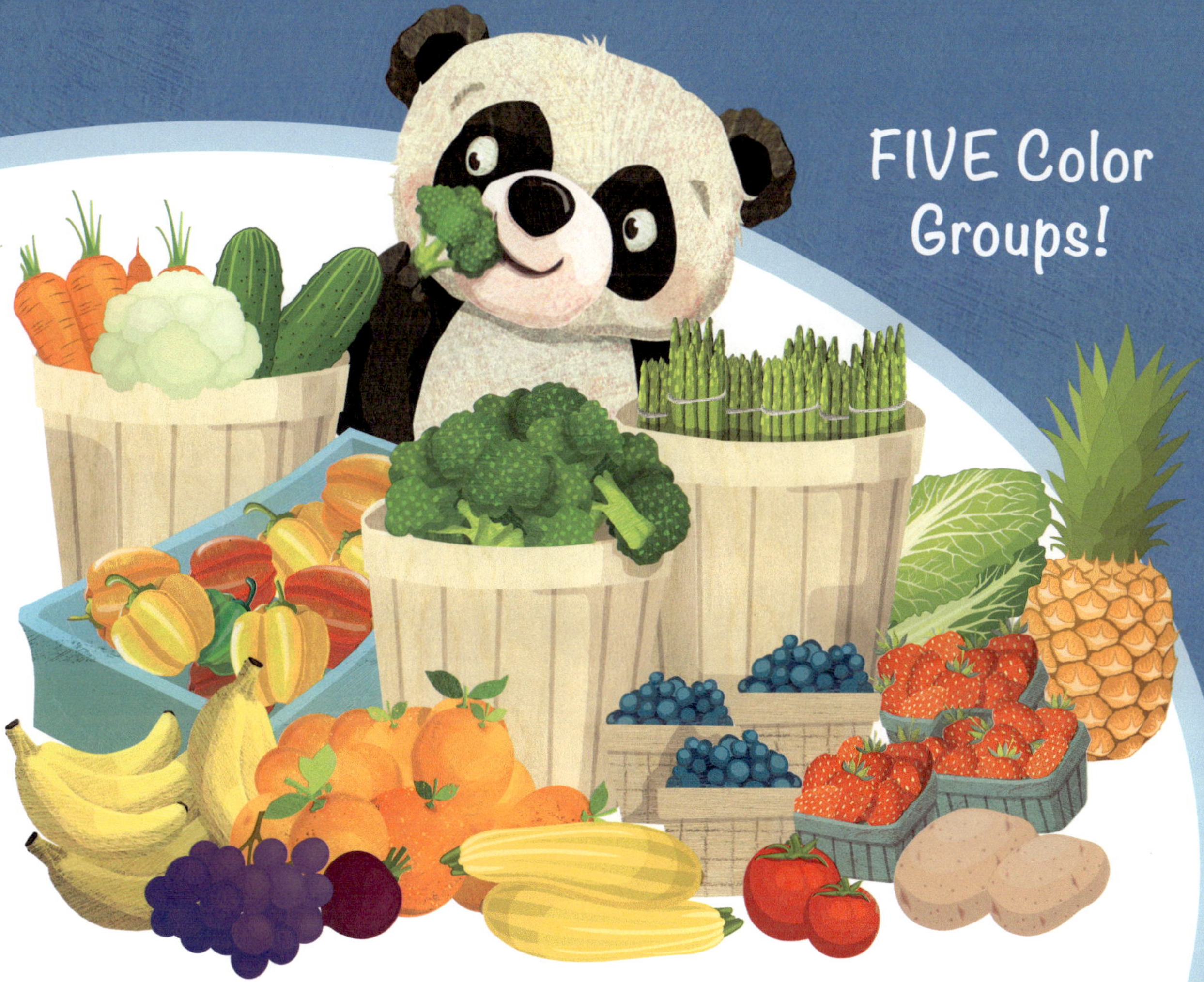

FIVE Color Groups!

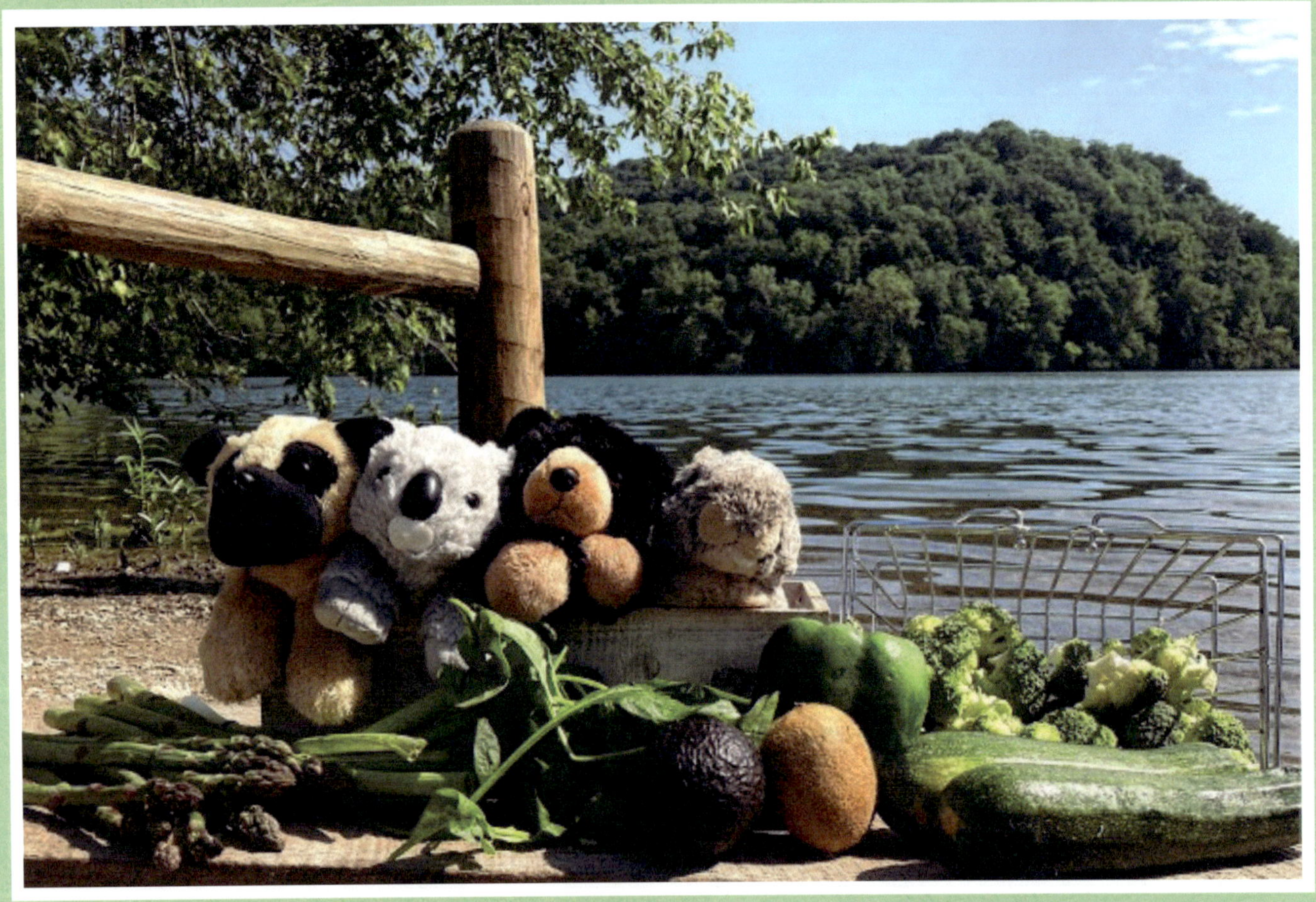

Boots the Bear eats

GREEN

fruits and veggies to help his body power-punch and fight against diseases.

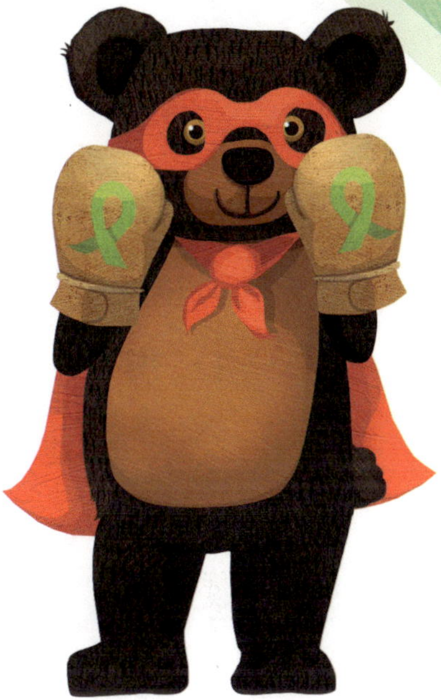

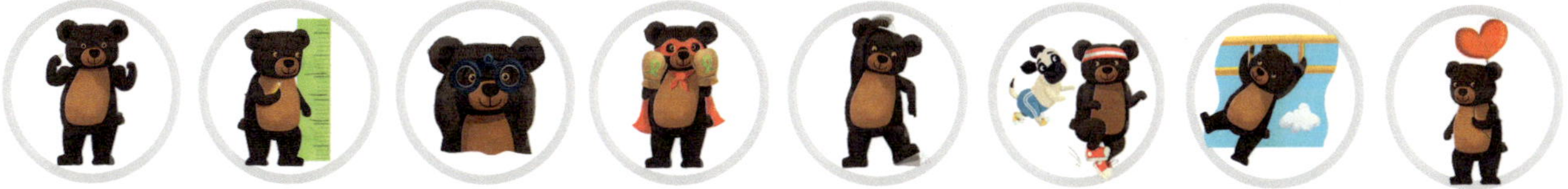

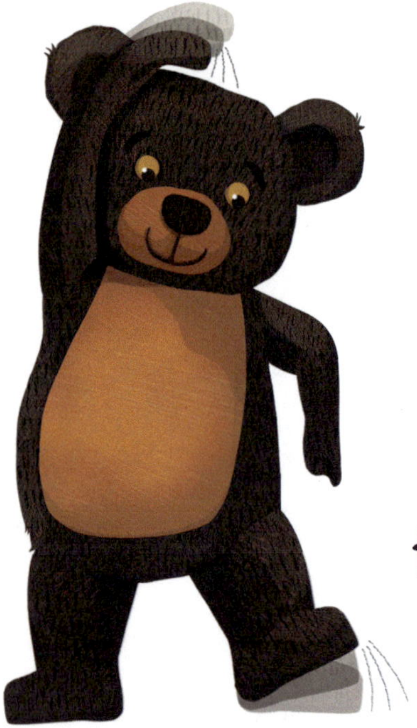

Boots the Bear eats

RED 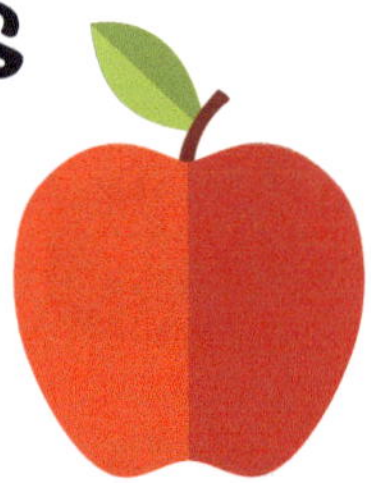

fruits and veggies because they help his body from head to shoulders and knees to toes.

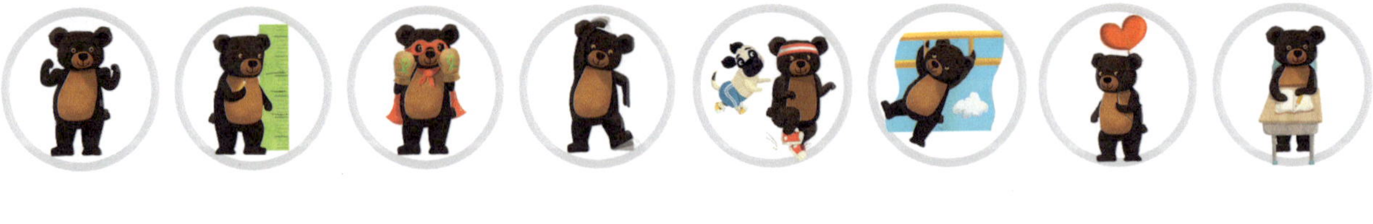

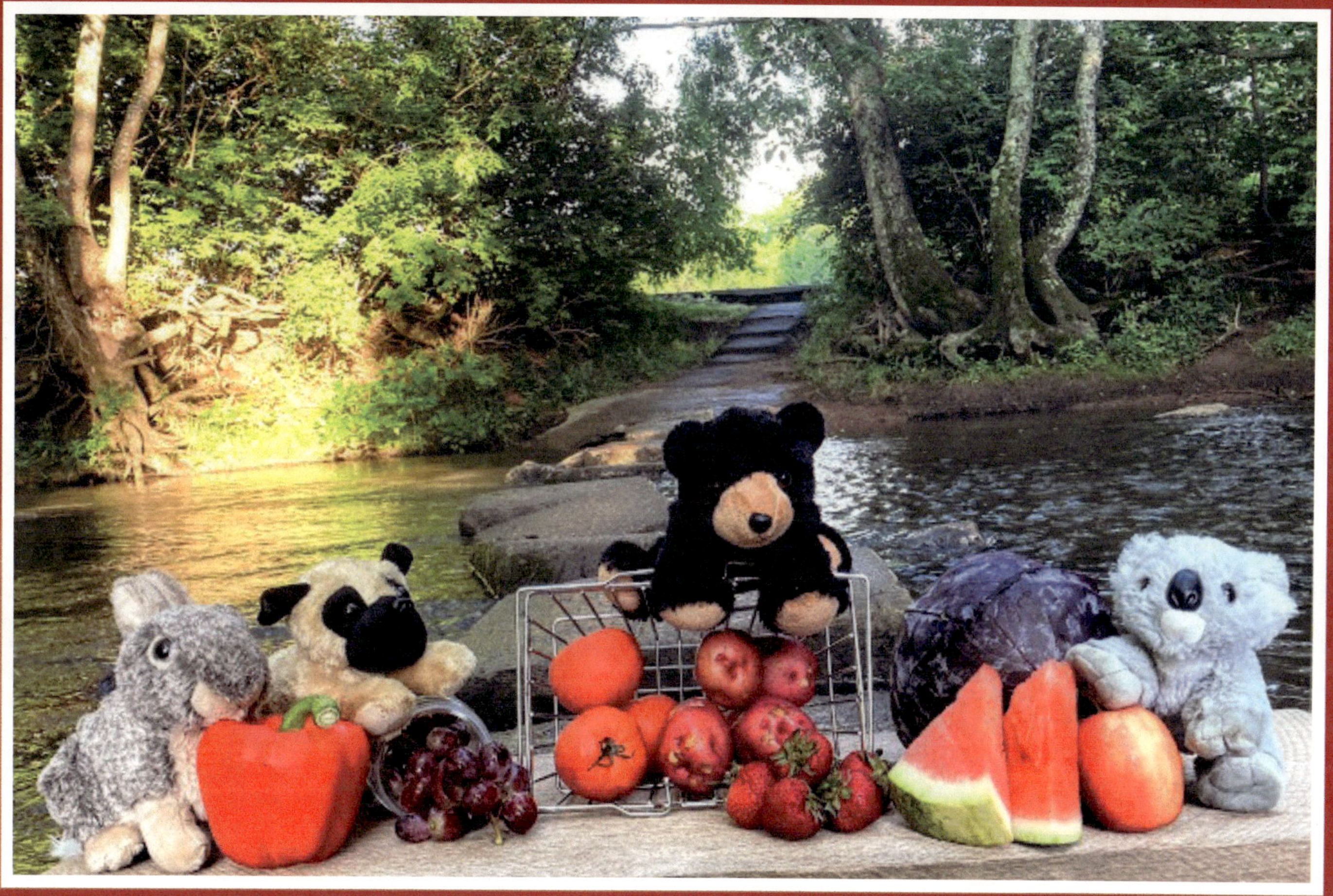

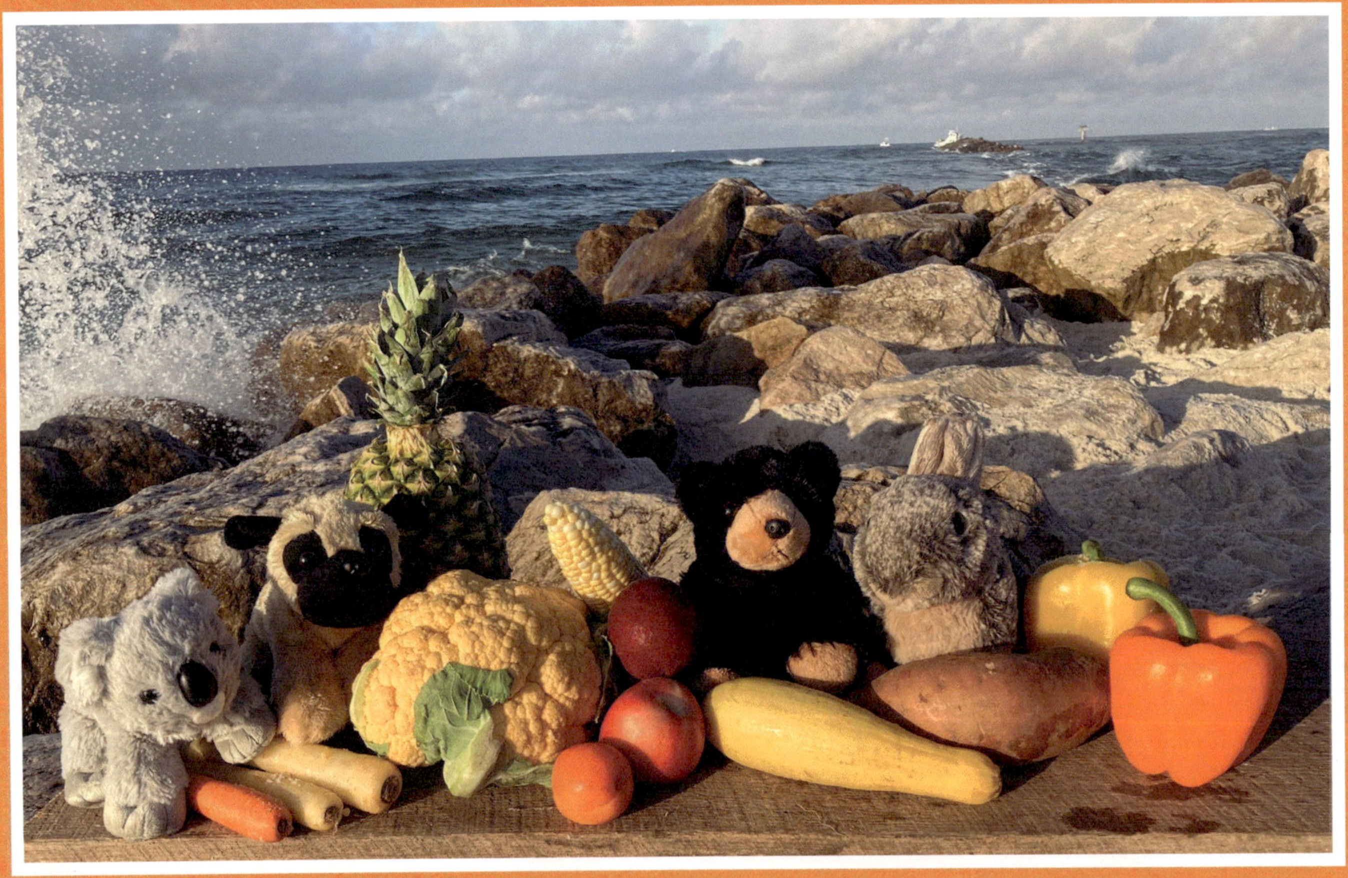

Boots the Bear eats

YELLOW & ORANGE

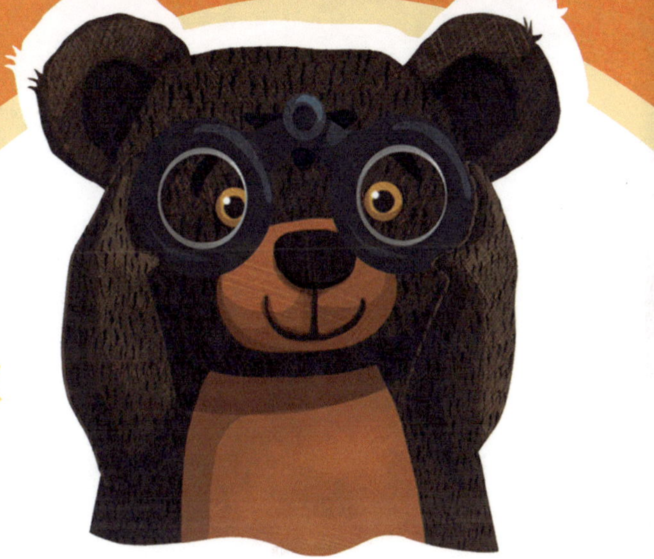

fruits and veggies because they help with super-sight and super-speed.

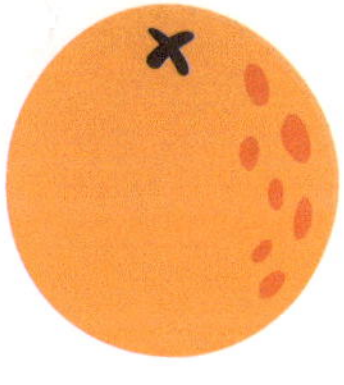

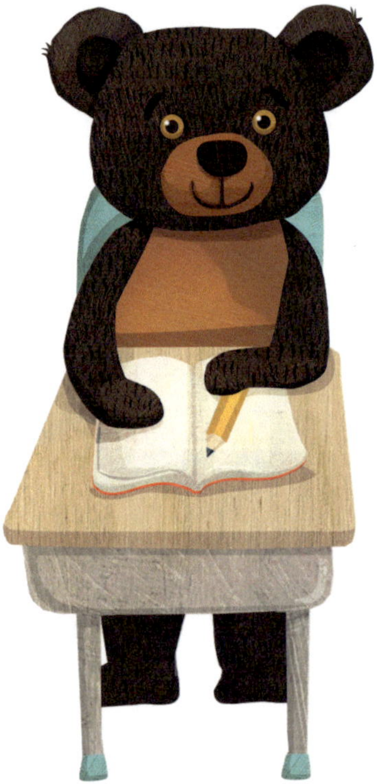

Boots the Bear eats

BLUE & PURPLE

fruits and veggies to help him grow his mega-mind

and well body.

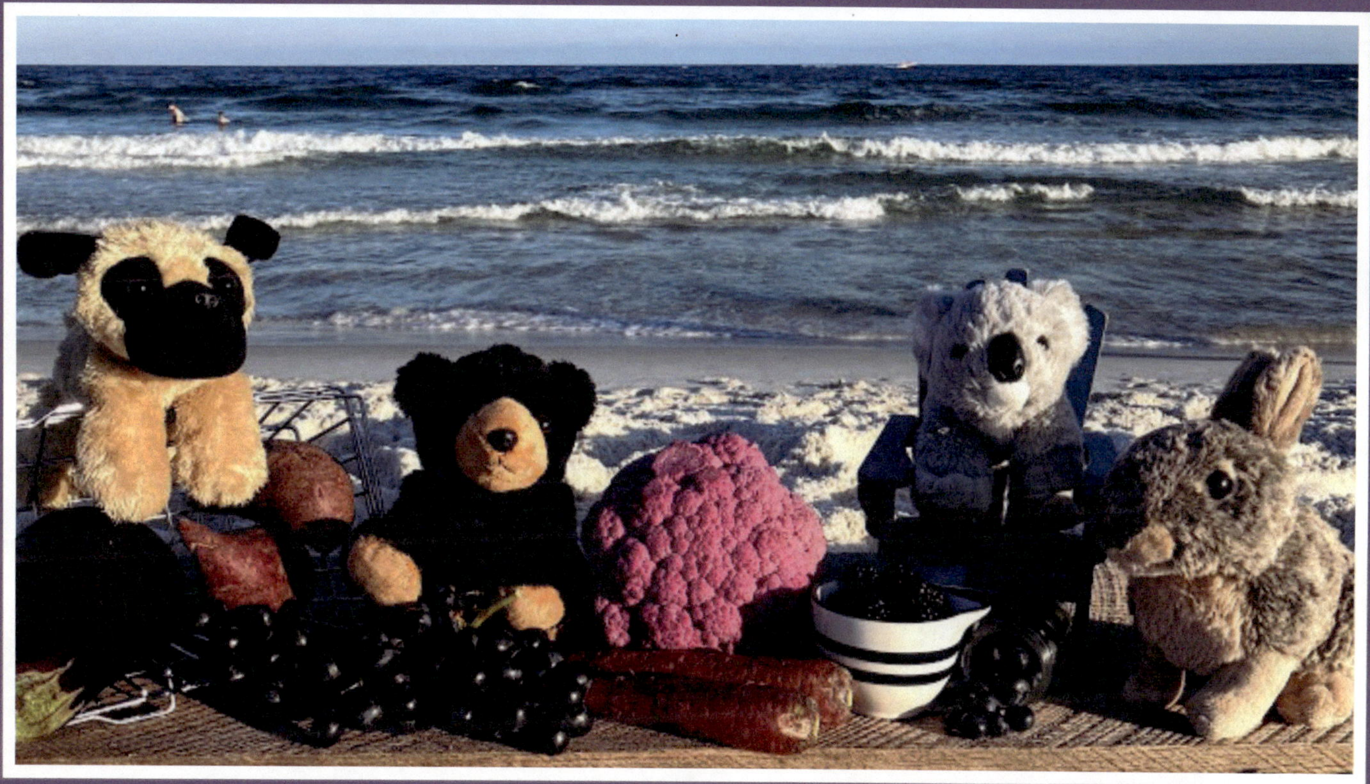

 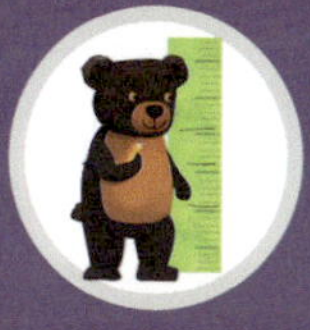   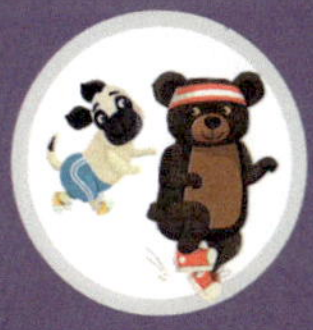   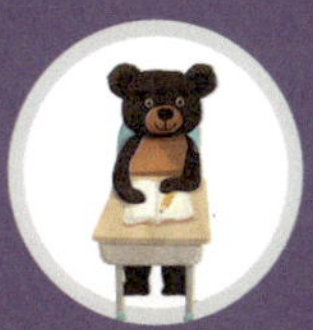

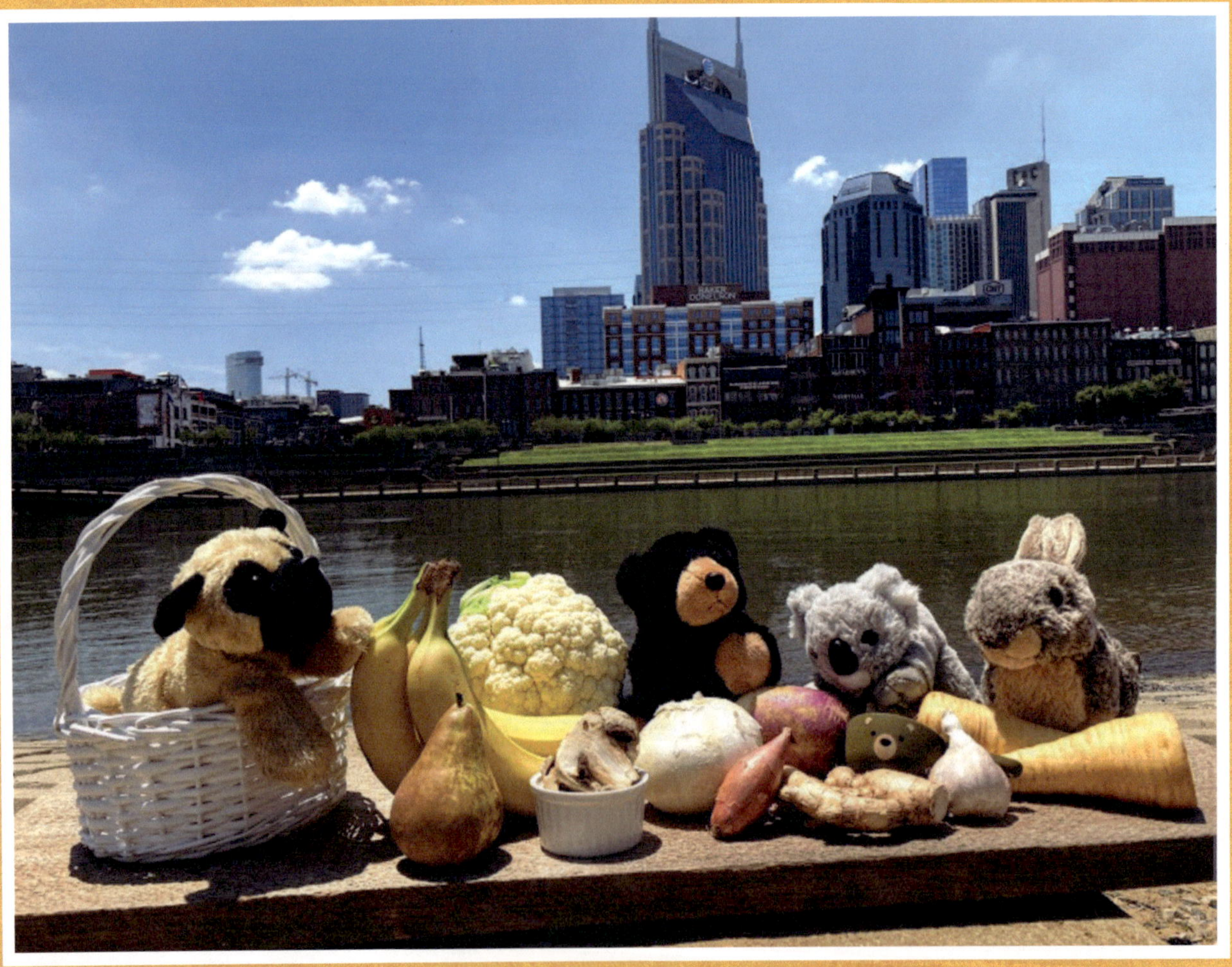

Boots the Bear eats

WHITE

fruits and veggies to help him be active, well, and fit.

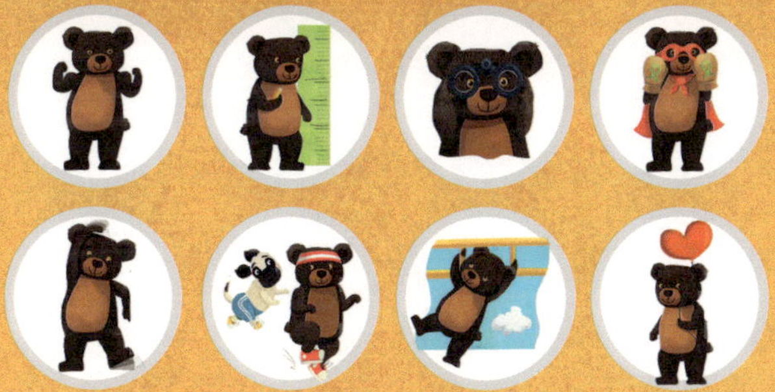

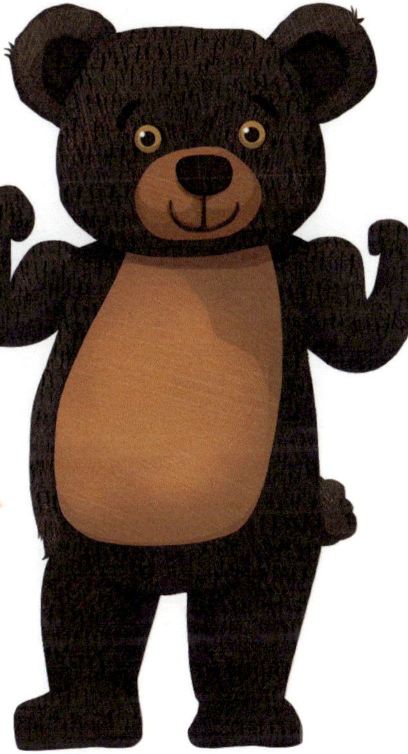

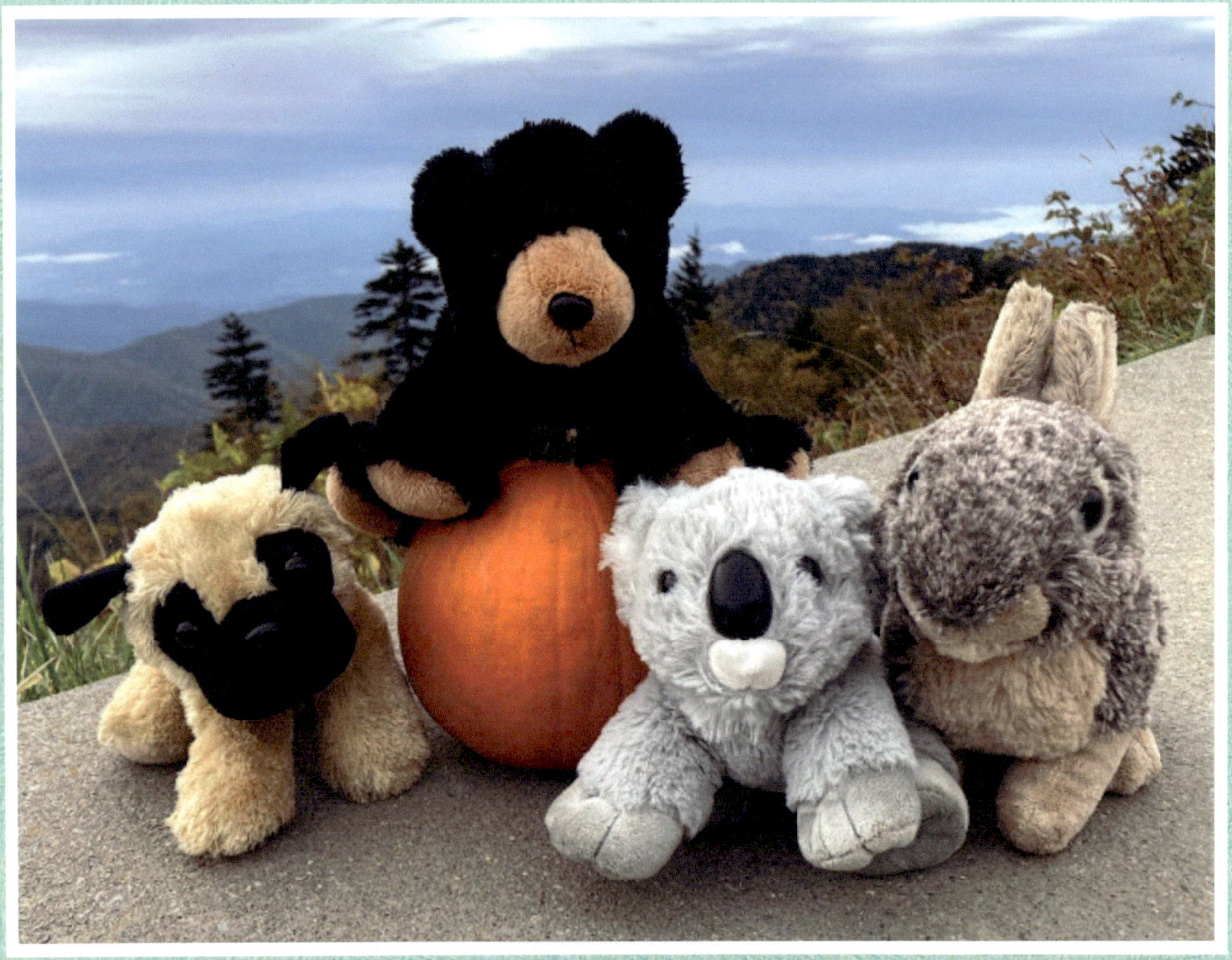

Boots the Bear asks,
"What will you eat to help
you run, play, and grow?"

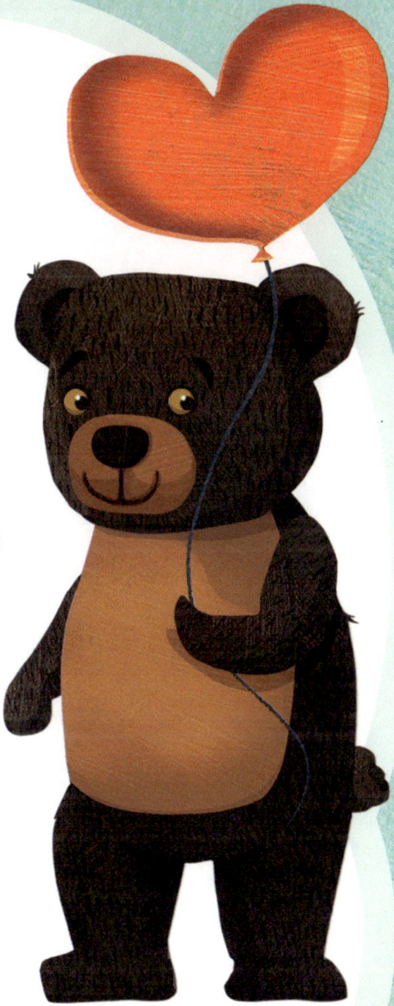

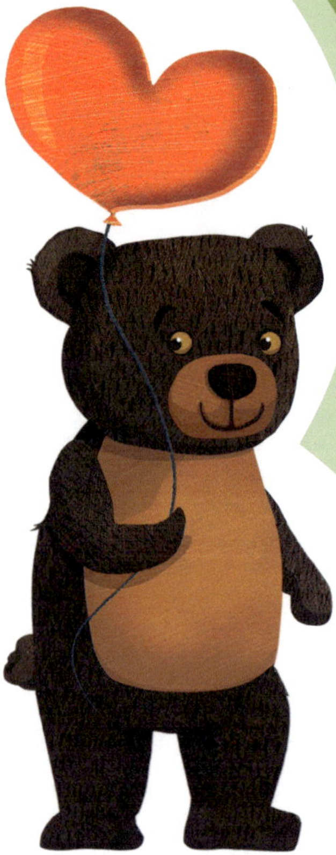

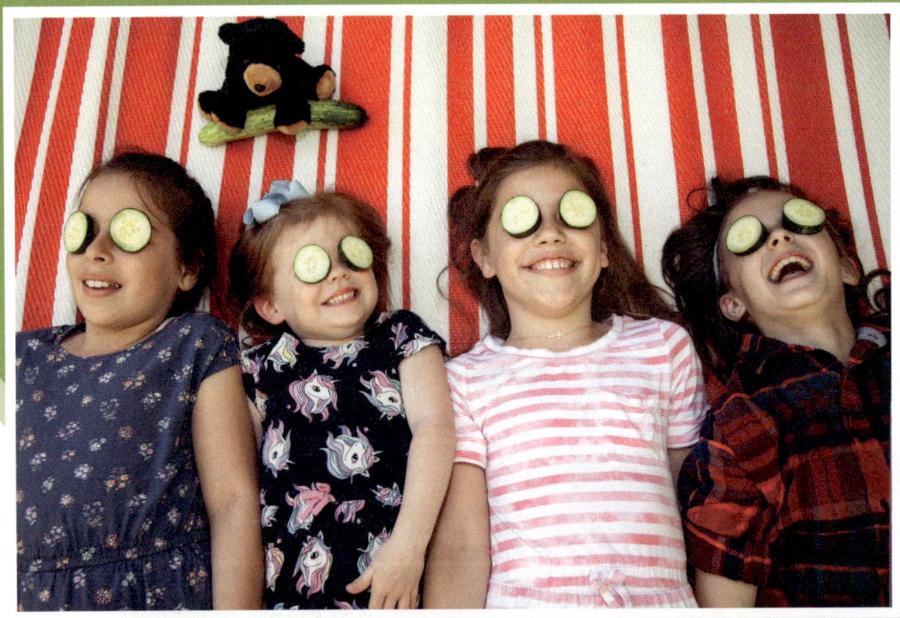

www.kidssunnybites.com

Made in United States
Troutdale, OR
11/03/2026

56844642R00055